EASY KETO

A Practical Approach to Lose Weight, Boost Health, Heal Your Body, and Regain Confidence in yourself

Alex Collins

CONTENTS

ABOUT THE BOOK

This book teaches so much on starting the ketogenic diet for dummies, starting the ketogenic diet can be overwhelming, so much to learn and so many resources to choose from. This book makes it very easy for dummies to carry out ketogenic diet without any contradiction. You will get exactly what you want to make keto surprisingly simple with meal plans, shopping lists, support, and lots more.

INTRODUCTION

The name "ketogenic diet" comes from the fact that the diet causes the production of small energy molecules called "ketones" or "ketone bodies". It is an alternative body fuel that is used when there is a lack of sugar (glucose) in the blood.Ketones are produced when you eat too few carbons (which break down very quickly into blood sugar) and only moderate amounts of protein (too much protein can also be converted to blood sugar).

Ketones are produced in the liver from fat. They are later used as energy throughout the body, including the brain. The brain is a very energy-consuming organ every day, and cannot feed directly on fat. Only works with glucose ... or ketones.

On a ketogenic diet, the entire body changes its energy supply to work almost exclusively with fat all the time. Insulin levels are reduced and fat burning increases dramatically. It is easy to access your body fat stores to burn them off. Of course, this is wonderful if you are trying to lose weight, but there are also other less obvious benefits, such as feeling less hungry and achieving a steady supply of energy.When the body produces ketones, it is said to be in ketosis. The quickest way to do this is to fast, not to eat anything - but obviously you cannot fast forever.

A ketogenic diet, on the other hand, can be consumed indefinitely and also results in ketosis. It brings many of the benefits of fasting - including weight loss - without having to fast.

The ketogenic diet, in all its variants, should be performed only under medical control and for a limited time only with menus that include an average percentage of protein combined with natural fat foods (butter, coconut oil, olive oil, pork fat, cream) and a low carbohydrate level.

Before talking about how the ketogenic diet is made, it is necessary to know how the combination of foods that make up each menu works and, above all, to understand that glucose, the simplest molecule to convert and use as energy, is always the chosen one. through the body before the rest of the existing options.

When glucose is used as the main source of energy, the body stores fat as a reserve and the more carbohydrates are consumed, the more blood glucose increases. If more protein and natural fats are consumed, the body adapts and changes its way of getting energy. Instead of using glucose, it uses body fat as a source of energy, leading to weight loss.

To make a ketogenic diet, you need to plan your daily menu, taking into account that most dishes should be made up of natural fats, protein, and a low amount of carbohydrate-providing foods. Between the main meals and as a snack, you can eat cheese or a handful of almonds.

It is important to remember that not all fats are equal. Thus, natural fats like olive oil, coconut oil or avocado provide health benefits, while the "trans fats" found in hamburger meat, margarine and all fried foods should be avoided as they are harmful to health.

01

ORIGIN OF KETOGENIC DIET

This diet initially emerged as a treatment for patients suffering from diabetes, a disease where the body of the person produces excess glucose, that is, the sugar present in their blood and even in their urine, basically due to a malfunction of the hormone in charge of insulin production.

With evidence that has been present since ancient times, even mentioned in stories from the Bible, where before Jesus was brought a child who presented manifestations of a convulsive condition and for which, Jesus himself recommended prayer and fasting. This being precisely the point we wish to reach; The word fast.

That it is the origin of the word Ketosis, which is mainly defined as a physiological effect caused in people by fasting; considered a deficit of the carbohydrates present in the body, which leads to using the burning or consumption of the fats present as a provider of the energy needed to live.

In the 1900s, an explorer named William Stephenson, studied the feeding of the indigenous Inuits of the Arctic regions, who were eaters of raw meat and fish, which caught the attention of this explorer, thinking that this food would cause them the disease called scurvy, a disease due to deficiencies of vitamin C in the body.

Which was not so since it was discovered, that this type of condition was only manifested when their diet was also accompanied by carbohydrates. Thus giving rise to a diet low in carbohydrate-containing foods for the following years by Robert Atkins, who was a cardiologist with overweight problems.

Dr. Atkins tried this diet initially with him and then with many of his patients, which was a complete success. However, at the time it was something that defied all the scientific beliefs of the moment, being considered therefore harmful to health, since it was considered that fats caused heart disease.In the year 1921 an endocrine doctor named Henry Rawle Geyelin, discovers this form of food and transforms it into a diet to be followed by people, in order to consume proteins and fats but eliminate carbohydrates and sugars.

This for the year of 1970, brings nutritional problems that caused deaths. Which was subsequently shown that it was not due to diet, because cholesterol did not rise, on the contrary, a decrease was observed, better than with many other diets. That is why the Ketogenic diet is not a hunger diet, it is a change in diet.

Thus, this form of radical, but effective, diet is also called Keto diet, since its name in English is Ketogenic. Where the human body begins to function as if it were a machine to burn fat. Which allows weight loss, and with it the improvement of health and greater physical performance.

The Ketogenic diet or Keto diet consists in the suppression, almost completely, of carbohydrates, which makes fats the energy nutrient to be used. By suppressing hydrates and using fats as a source of energy, you enter a state called ketosis, or what is the same, the number of ketones in the blood rises. This state is similar to what the body experiences when it is fasting motivated by moments of rest, be it a nap or nighttime sleep.

Numerous studies such as the one published in the prestigious journal Cell Metabolism open the hope that ketogenic diets not only reduce weight, eating in a satiating and healthy way, but that they seem to improve memory and life expectancy as it improves the profile Lipid by reducing triglyceride and total cholesterol levels, ketone bodies promote the absence of hunger, which promotes weight loss without the usual feeling of anxiety, thanks to the satiating power of proteins and fats, which they take longer to digest than hydrates.

What Is A Ketogenic Diet

The ketogenic diet (or keto diet in its abbreviated form) is a low-carb, high-fat diet that offers many health benefits.In fact, about 20 studies show that this type of diet can help you lose weight and improve health.Ketogenic diets can have benefits even against diabetes, cancer, epilepsy and Alzheimer's.

What is a ketogenic diet?

The ketogenic diet is a low-carb, high-fat diet that shares many similarities with Atkins and low-carb diets.This diet involves drastically reducing carbohydrates and replacing them with fats. This decrease exposes the body to a metabolic state called ketosis.When this happens, the body becomes incredibly efficient and can convert all fat into energy. It also converts fat to ketones within the liver, which can provide more energy to the brain.Ketogenic diets may cause reductions in blood sugar and insulin levels. This, along with the increase in ketones, offers numerous health benefits.

There are many versions of ketogenic diets, including:

- The Standard Ketogenic Diet (ECD): It is a very low carbohydrate diet with moderate protein and high fat intake. Includes 75% fat, 20% protein and only 5% carbohydrates.

- A cyclic ketogenic diet (CHD): This plan involves higher carbohydrate refills, for example, 5 straight ketogenic days for 2 carbohydrate days.

- Adapted ketogenic diet (DCA): allows you to add carbohydrates on training days.

- A high protein ketogenic diet: Similar to a standard ketogenic diet, but includes more protein. Normal is 60% fat, 35% protein and 5% carbohydrate.

However, only standard and high protein ketogenic diets have been thoroughly studied. Cyclic or adapted diets are more advanced methods and are mainly used by athletes or bodybuilders.A ketogenic diet is an effective way to lose weight and lower risk factors in some diseases.

In fact, research shows that the ketogenic diet exceeds the normally recommended low-fat diets.Also, the goal of the diet is that you can lose weight without counting calories or keeping track of your intake.One study found that people on a ketogenic diet lose 2.2 times more weight than those calories and fat. Triglyceride and HDL cholesterol levels also show improvement.Another study found that people on ketogenic diets lose 3 times more weight than those traditionally recommended by Diabetes UK.There are many reasons why the ketogenic diet is better for the low fat diet such as increased protein intake which offers numerous benefits.Increasing ketones, lowering sugar levels, and improving insulin sensitivity may also play a key role.

Diabetes is characterized by changes in metabolism, increased blood sugar and decreased insulin functions.

The ketogenic diet can help you lose excess fat, which is closely related to type 2 diabetes, prediabetes and metabolic syndrome.One study found that the ketogenic diet improved insulin sensitivity by a huge 75% increase.In another study of people suffering from type 2 diabetes, it was found that 7 out of 21 participants were able to stop taking all diabetes medicines.In another study, the ketogenic group lost 11.4 kg (24.4 pounds), compared to 6.9 kg (15.2 pounds) than the high carbohydrate group lost. It is an important benefit if we consider the relationship between weight and type 2 diabetes.In addition, 95.2% of the ketogenic group was able to discontinue or reduce diabetes medications, compared with 62% of the high carbohydrate group.

The current ketogenic diet originated as a way to treat neurological diseases such as epilepsy.

Some studies have shown that diet can have benefits in a wide variety of diseases:

- Heart disease: Ketogenic diet may improve risk factors such as body fat, HDL cholesterol levels, blood pressure and blood sugar.
- Cancer: Currently, this diet has been used to treat many types of cancer and reduce the growth of tumors.
- Alzheimer's: Ketological diet can reduce the symptoms of the disease and slow its progression.
- Epilepsy: Research has shown that ketogenic dieting can greatly reduce epileptic seizures in children.
- Parkinson's: One study found that dieting helped improve Parkinson's symptoms.
- Polycystic Ovarian Syndrome: Ketogenic diet can help reduce insulin levels, which may play a key role in polycystic ovary syndrome.
- Brain Injury: An animal study found that diet can reduce concussions and help the patient recover after suffering these injuries.
- Acne: Reduced insulin levels and reduced sugar intake or processed foods can improve acne.

Foods to Avoid

Any high carbohydrate food should be avoided.

Below is a list of foods that should be reduced or eliminated in a ketogenic diet:

- Sugary foods: Soft drinks, fruit juices, smoothies, pies, ice cream, sweets, etc.
- Cereals or starches: products derived from wheat, rice, pasta, cereals, etc.
- Fruits: All fruits except small portions of fruits such as strawberries.
- Beans or vegetables: peas, red beans, lentils, chickpeas, etc.
- Root vegetables and tubers: potatoes, sweet potatoes, carrots, parsnips, etc.
- Dietary or low fat products: They are usually highly processed and high in carbohydrates.
- Some condiments or sauces: Above all, those that contain sugar and saturated fats.
- Saturated fats: limit intake of refined oils, mayonnaise, etc.
- Alcohol: Due to its high carbohydrate content, many alcoholic beverages should be eliminated in a ketogenic diet.
- Sugar-Free Diet Foods: They are usually high in sugar alcohols, which can affect ketone levels. These foods also tend to be highly processed.

Food to eat

You should base most meals around these foods:

- Meat: Red meat, steak, ham, sausage, bacon, chicken and turkey.
- Fatty fish: like salmon, trout, tuna and mackerel.
- Eggs: Look for pasteurized omega 3 rich eggs.
- Butter and Cream: If possible, look for foods that have been fed grass.
- Cheese: Unprocessed cheese (cheddar, goat, creamy, blue or mozzarella cheese).
- Nuts and seeds: almonds, walnuts, flax seeds, pumpkin seeds, chia seeds, etc.
- Healthy oils: Above all, extra virgin olive oil, coconut oil and avocado oil.
- Avocado: Whole avocados or guacamole made naturally.
- Low Carb Vegetables: Most green vegetables, tomatoes, onions and peppers, etc.
- Condiments: You can use salt, pepper, some healthy herbs and spices.

Contraindications

Studies have revealed that in general, this type of diet is usually good for all those who need it, either to lose weight or to improve their health in some way, however it is necessary that in the following cases, use the advice of a nutritionist before following her:

- Although the diet allows lowering sugar levels, which is a benefit for diabetics, if they are taking medications they should be under medical supervision, as they may need to lower their insulin levels.

- People who suffer from hypertension, need to take medications for their control, and following this diet may suffer alterations, although positive, that lead them to lower the dose of their medication, so they must be under medical supervision.

- Despite being an excellent way to lose weight for women who have given birth, and are breastfeeding, it is not recommended to take this diet, at least while you are administering breastfeeding to your baby, as its effect for He has not been determined.

At this point, it is important to clarify that there are still many controversies regarding the use of the Ketogenic diet, especially for people who consume medications, as they may require that their doses be changed, so our recommendation is always to consult with your doctor before starting any diet.

Experiences

There are people who have expressed their experience in the media, especially online and social networks; be some cases of people who testify that in the face of conditions such as hyperthyroidism, they need the use of medications such as Eutirox, which controls the functioning of their thyroid.

But despite this they constantly gain weight and the only way they have been able to control it is by using the Ketogenic

Diet, and seeing that they can lose weight with it and control their condition, they have maintained it for as long as possible ; the person managed to lose 3.5 kilos in three weeks and feels positive to continue carrying it.

Does the Ketogenic Diet work?

The evidence has shown so far that the Ketogenic Diet does work. Due to the fact that it allows fats to be burned, is used to provide the energy that your body needs and not supplying carbohydrates, you will not gain weight, but on the contrary, you can lose it, in a fast, effective and safe way.

Well, sugars are no longer supplied to the body, which is what increases blood glucose levels. Being these sugars full of calories, and by suppressing them the body uses the energy produced by fats, which is beneficial.

On the other hand, the consumption of healthy fats allows people to feel full when eating, and thereby reduce their need to be consuming large amounts of meals, as well as having to peck between one meal and another, which benefits their loss of weight.

Results

The results have been verified by comparative studies of diets high in carbohydrates and the Ketogenic Diet, where carbohydrate consumption is low; following studies has stated that this group carbohydrate consumption is low, so it had a better performance to lose weight.

Where they burned about 250 calories more than people who followed carbohydrate diets. Considering the scientists that the people of the Ketogenic Diet, have had to consume more calories than the other group and thus have lost weight.

How much do you get off?

This is a topic that is usually very variable, due to the personal condition presented by people, as for many of them, there are foods that can make them gain more weight than other people who consume the same foods.

Everything also depends on the overweight that each person has, as well as the fact that they do any physical activity or not. But especially the metabolism of the person who wishes to follow the diet.

But it is estimated that one and a half kilograms per week can be lost on average. However, for people who have more accumulated fat, they can lose up to four kilos weekly. The general rule is that as long as the person has less body mass, weight loss will take place more slowly.

02

THE BENEFITS OF A KETOGENIC DIET

The benefits of a ketogenic diet are similar to those of other low carbohydrate diets, but are much more effective than more liberal low carbohydrate diets. You can think of the ketogenic diet as a low-carb, extremely effective diet that maximizes benefits.

Lose weight

Turning your body into a fat-burning machine has clear benefits for weight loss. Fat burning increases dramatically, while insulin levels - the fat-storage hormone - drop dramatically. This creates ideal conditions for losing body fat without starving. About 20 leading-edge scientific studies show that, compared to other diets, ketogenic, low-carbohydrate diets cause weight loss more effectively.

Appetite control

By following a ketogenic diet, you take the reins of your appetite. When the body burns fat all the time, it has constant access to an amount of stored energy equivalent to consuming several weeks or even several months. This drastically reduces the feeling of hunger. It is a very common experience and studies show it.

Eating less and losing weight becomes much easier - just don't eat until you are hungry. This greatly facilitates the practice of intermittent fasting, which intensifies the correction of type 2 diabetes and accelerates weight loss. Plus, you'll save a lot of time and money when you no longer have to eat snacks all the time. Many people just feel the need to eat twice a day (often skipping breakfast), and others only eat once.

Not having to fight hunger also has the potential to help with problems like sugar or food addiction and possibly certain eating disorders such as bulimia. Only by feeling satiated can you solve part of the problem. Food can stop being an enemy and become your friend - or simply feed your body. What you prefer.

Constant energy and greater mental focus

Ketosis results in a steady flow of energy (ketones) to the brain and thus prevents major ups and downs in blood sugar. This often causes an improvement in mental focus and concentration.Many people use ketogenic diets specifically to increase their mental performance. Also, many people notice an increase in their energy levels while in ketosis.When you are adapted to the ketogenic diet, the brain does not need carbohydrates. It feeds on ketones all the time, which is the perfect fuel for mental focus and energy.

Blood glucose control and correction of type 2 diabetes

A ketogenic diet controls blood glucose levels and is excellent for reversing type 2 diabetes. This has been shown in scientific studies. It makes sense because the keto diet lowers blood sugar and reduces the negative effect of high insulin levels.

Improvements in health markers

There are many studies showing that low carbohydrate diets improve important health markers including cholesterol profile (HDL and triglycerides), blood glucose, insulin levels and blood pressure.These markers that usually improve following a ketogenic diet are linked to the so-called "metabolic syndrome" and improvements in body weight, waist circumference, type 2 diabetes, etc.

Reduction of digestive problems

Ketogenic diet can calm the stomach, causing less gas, less cramps and pain, etc.For many people, this is the biggest benefit of eating keto, and it usually only takes 1-2 days to observe.

An increase in physical endurance

Ketogenic diets can greatly increase stamina by providing constant access to all energy stored in body fat. The supply of stored carbohydrates (glycogen) lasts only a few hours of intense exercise, or even less. But your fat stores contain enough energy to easily last weeks or even months.

Epilepsy

Ketogenic diet is a proven medical treatment to combat epilepsy and has been used since the 1920s. Traditionally, it has been used in children but has recently been successfully tested in adults as well. Using a ketogenic diet as a treatment for epilepsy may reduce the need for anticonvulsant medications and even prevent seizures. This reduces the side effects of medications, improving mental performance.

Consequences of the Keto Diet

We can mention some cons of the ketogenic diet since it is not suitable for everyone, it is advisable to consult with a healthcare professional before starting this diet, to avoid complications.

- Its contribution of vitamins, minerals, and fiber is very low, greatly limits the intake of fruits and vegetables.
- It can generate episodes of constipation and other adverse effects such as cramping, halitosis or asthenia.

- Obsession can develop to maintain the state of ketosis which can cause a loss of muscle mass.
- It can end up consuming too much and not losing any weight, while the body can develop insulin resistance.
- You have to be careful with this diet: "If done incorrectly you can modify the parameters of lipids in the blood, which would endanger our health."

KETOGENIC DIET PHASES

During the early phase, when the body goes into a state of ketosis, some mild symptoms may occur, although they disappear quickly:

- indigestion,
- Constipation,
- fatigue,
- Difficulty concentrating,
- headache or
- insomnia.

Breathing can smell like acetone exhaling its toxins. It is characteristic of ketosis and ketogenic diets.

How can I measure ketosis?

Ketosis can be detected in blood, urine and even air.

The cheapest and simplest way is to urine through test strips that are sold in drugstores. However, the concentration of ketone bodies and their elimination in the urine tend to decrease over time, as your body makes better use of them as a source of energy.

This is why the most accurate way is through blood tests. Blood test strips similar to those used by diabetics are also sold.

To avoid the reduction in muscle mass that can be caused by weight loss by following a weight loss diet, you need to keep your protein intake close to 35% and exercise. This will maintain your body's muscle mass and may even increase it, unlike other diets.

From time to time, with the frequency suggested by the specialist (doctor or nutritionist), the amount of carbohydrates should be increased, but taking into account that in the first two or three months the diet should be more rigorous.

On the other hand, you should keep in mind that a severe dietary restriction may reduce quality of life and that the answer to some questions, such as the long-term side effects of ketogenic diet, is unknown.

PRINCIPLES AND EXAMPLES

To understand the principles of the Ketogenic Diet, you must start our knowledge with what is ketosis, being called the situation that you want to generate in our body, with the diet, something that has been considered to the situation of the organism when it is fasting. This is done when we undergo an insufficient supply of food, or when we follow a diet that has dietary restrictions especially in terms of carbohydrates, represented by carbohydrates and saccharides, which are nothing other than sugars.Given the lack of this type, the body produces energy molecules, which are called ketones, considered as alternative energy, which gives the body the necessary contributions to cover the faults of the carbohydrates, which are precisely those that generate blood sugar.

When a person consumes few carbohydrates, ketones are produced at the liver level and caused by fats, being used to give energy to the brain and the whole body. But it is important to consider that our brain does not feed directly on fats, it does it from glucose and its lack of ketones.

A ketogenic diet (keto) is a very low carb diet, which converts the body into a fat-burning machine. It has many potential benefits for weight loss, health, and performance, but also some possible initial side effects.

A ketogenic diet is similar to other low carb diets, such as the Atkins diet or LCHF (low carb, high fat). These diets often end up being ketogenic more or less by accident. The main difference between strict LCHF and ketogenic is that the protein is restricted in the second.

A ketogenic diet is specifically designed to result in ketosis. It is possible to measure and adapt to achieve optimal ketone levels for health, weight loss or for physical and mental performance. You can then learn how to use this diet to achieve your personal goals.Here are the typical foods to enjoy a ketogenic diet. The numbers are net carbohydrates per 100 grams. To remain in ketosis, in general, less is better:

Low Carb and Ketogenic Foods

The most important thing to achieve ketosis is to avoid eating most carbohydrates. You probably need to keep your carbohydrate intake at less than 50 grams per day of net carbohydrates, ideally below 20 grams.

This means that you will have to completely avoid sugary sweet foods, in addition to starchy foods such as bread, pasta, rice, and potatoes. Basically, follow the guidelines for a strict low carb diet, and remember that it is supposed to be high in fat, not high in protein. An approximate guideline is below 10% of energy in carbohydrates (fewer carbohydrates, more effective), 15-25% protein (the lower end is more effective) and 70% or more fat.

03

The Basics Of Ketogenic Diet

It is important to note that the fact that people have different metabolism, genetic tendencies and levels of physical activity makes it possible to enter ketosis with different proportions of macronutrients.

(Macronutrients are carbohydrates, proteins and fats.)

However, a traditional ketogenic diet recommendation would summarize the following proportions:

- Carbohydrate intake not exceeding 5 to 10% of total calories;

- Protein intake is about 20 to 30% of total calories consumed daily;

- And fat intake provides 65-75% of calories - possibly even more.

(1 gram of carbohydrate has 4 calories, 1 gram of protein has 4 calories and 1 gram of fat has 9 calories).

In this case, the amount of carbohydrate we refer to above is liquid carbohydrate - which is nothing more than the total amount of carbohydrate in a food minus the amount of fiber.

How to Start a 5-Step Ketogenic Diet

The 5 steps are as follows - and we'll talk more about each one below:

- Start with the macronutrient division detailed above;
- Take body measurements and body photos;
- Try for at least 4 weeks;
- After 4 weeks, measure progress again;
- Evaluate and adjust as needed.

Step 1 to Follow a Successful Ketogenic Diet - Obey the Macronutrient Ratio: The Fat, Protein, and Carbohydrate Ratio

This step is critical for beginners in the ketogenic diet. This is because most beginners of the ketone diet do not have the exact notion of what to eat and what not to eat. In this scenario, it is very important to understand well what proportion of macronutrients (carbohydrates, protein, fat) you should eat.

In the low-carb ketogenic diet, the proportion of macronutrients is approximately as follows:

- fat: 60% to 75% of daily calories;
- protein: 15% to 25% daily calories;
- Carbohydrates: 5% to 10% of daily calories.

And you don't have to worry about calories now: let's use the proportion of the traditional ketogenic diet - which should have benefits like increased satiety and insulin sensitivity - which in themselves should start to improve caloric intake. So don't worry: just follow the macronutrients of the ketogenic diet and eat until you are satisfied with each meal.

Step 2 to Successfully Follow a Ketogenic Diet - Take Body Measurements and Body Photos

When embarking on a new project, we are often excited to do everything right and achieve the results we so desire.Over time, however, this initial excitement can usually subside - especially if we feel we are not making much progress.

Therefore, to keep motivation high and get objective data to gauge where your progress is going, it is important to be able to measure your results.These steps, along with before-and-after photos, are powerful indicators that you're headed in the right direction and help keep you through even the most boring moments of the weight loss process.And we know that a lot of people don't like to take shirtless photos when they are overweight - after all, they don't feel good about their bodies and they don't want to have that record.But it's worth it: after all, it's the "before" image that you'll use to compare it to your current moment.

Step 3 to follow a successful ketogenic diet - try for at least 4 weeks

We will not expand this much much simply because there is not much to say.Just ask: please don't be one of those people who starts a diet and follows it for 3 days.Change does not happen overnight.Think about how many days, months, years your body has taken to stay in shape.I am sure it was not just 4 weeks.Therefore, you will certainly need time to get good results.And we know that at the beginning it can be hard to believe that you will have results.After all, with the ketogenic diet, you'll lose weight feeling good - because you're not hungry, you don't have to eat every three hours and you can taste delicious recipes - and that seems contrary to everything you've ever heard out there. all your life!Therefore, to be comfortable during the ketogenic diet, it is important to understand that there is science behind it - and to trust the process.Therefore, we recommend that you follow the diet for at least 4 weeks before attempting to evaluate results and deciding whether or not this diet is appropriate.

Important: If you have a known health problem (such as diabetes, hypertension, or any other illness), talk to a trusted doctor before you even start your diet - including because you may need to make adjustments to your medication dosages as diet can help to control diabetes and liver steatosis.

Step 4 to successfully follow a ketogenic diet - after 4 weeks, measure progress again

This is a straightforward step and it's about you measuring progress at predetermined intervals - preferably under conditions as similar as possible.For example, on the same day of the week, at the same time, at the same time of the menstrual cycle for women .And of course, never measure progress right after a day of rubbish.

Step 5 to Successfully Follow a Ketogenic Diet - Evaluate and Adjust as Needed

This point is optional if you want to make adjustments to best suit the diet to your lifestyle.After all, for most people, a ketogenic diet can cause fat burning even without exercise and not counting calories.This is because, as we explained earlier, in the ketogenic diet you will train your body to use fat as a form of food rather than carbohydrate.But if you want to adjust your diet for results, you can count on the help of exercise, control your total calorie intake, add some form of intermittent fasting, or even modify the proportion of macronutrients to meet your goals. Remembering that it is often important to consult with a professional focused on low carbohydrate philosophy to understand the best way to make these adjustments.

Since we talked about adjusting macronutrient intake, we are referring to what we saw in step 1:

- 5-10% of total calories from carbohydrates;

- 20-30% of total calories from protein;
- 65-75% of total calories from fat.

However, many people do not like to keep counting all the nutrients until exhaustion.This is because there are three easier alternatives that we will explore now, so you can decide how best to enter and stay in ketosis.

#1 Alternative to Ketogenic Diet - Control Carbohydrate Intake Only and Let the Rest of the Diet Fit For You

This is because by controlling your carbohydrate intake, you will have to automatically increase your fat intake to maintain your satiety - to increase your chances of getting into nutritional ketosis.So you just have to be careful to eat low carbohydrate foods and supplement the rest of the diet with good protein and fat.

And that is why it is important not to starve to this diet - as this ensures that you are providing your body with the right and proper fuel for its functioning (in this case, good fats).Part of the reason this method is so good is that in nature we often find protein associated with fat.That is, most cuts of meat, eggs, chickens and more contain no protein in isolation.Therefore, by maintaining protein intake and decreasing carbohydrate intake, you naturally tend to increase your fat intake to compensate.And to succeed in this approach, the instruction is simple enough: You don't have to be obsessed with finding out how much fat is in each food, just don't escape the natural fat in foods that everything should adjust automatically.In other words: eat eggs with yolk, fry butter or lard foods, eat chicken skin and fat (or choose fatter cuts).(Interestingly, it is this ability to reduce carbohydrate consumption by using only a few processed foods that often a paleolithic diet can also be considered ketogenic - that is, a real food-based diet can also induce nutritional ketosis.).And even if you end up increasing your protein intake a little, this should not be a problem.

First, there are already several studies proving that a high protein diet does not cause damage or stress to the liver or kidneys in healthy individuals.

(For those who already have problems with these organs, it is interesting to consult a qualified professional.)

And second, why is there a debate about protein limitation in a ketogenic diet - and that we detail in our full text "Is there too much protein in the ketogenic diet? "

For now, all you need to know to properly follow this # 1 alternative is:

- Limit carbohydrate intake (many people opt for 20 to 30 g of liquid carbohydrate per day, sometimes even less);
- Eat to satiety;
- Do not run away from the natural fat of foods.

Alternative # 2 to Maintain Ketogenic Diet - Controlling Nutrient Intake with the Help of Applications

Ecology is really a wonderful thing.Thanks to her, we were able to access incredible scientific studies, listen to the advice of top-level debate experts, and convey the best food information.And one of my favorite uses of technology is being able to rely on mobile apps to control nutrient intake when I'm on a ketogenic diet.One of the most popular among our readers is Fat Secret, because it's easy to see information and set goals for calories, nutrients and even liquid carbohydrates.

Alternative # 3 to Maintain Ketogenic Diet - Eat Only Allowed Foods

If you have read this far, you already understand that the idea behind the ketogenic diet or ketone diet is simply to induce the state of ketosis in your body by making fat burning easier.And to help you stay in this state, there are the two alternatives above - controlling nutrient intake to facilitate ketosis entry and maintenance.However, you don't have to be obsessed with controlling everything you eat - and in fact for many people it's even counterproductive.In this case, only eat only foods that naturally already have the proportion of macronutrients we are trying to reach.That is, low carbohydrate, moderate protein and high fat foods.

MENU - EXAMPLE 7 DAYS OF KETOGENIC DIET

This is an example of a week's menu for anyone following a ketogenic diet plan.It provides less than 30 grams of total carbs per day.

Monday

- Breakfast: Omelet with assorted vegetables.
- Lunch: Kebabs with lettuce and tomato salad.
- Dinner: Braised chicken drumstick and nutritious cabbage soup.

Tuesday

- Breakfast: Bacon and Eggs.
- Lunch: Ground beef with zucchini and mixed salad (leaves, tomato, cucumber).
- Dinner: Low-carb eggplant lasagna or what's left of other meals.

Wednesday

- Breakfast: Low carb cheese.
- Lunch: Butter-fried pork chop and stir-fried vegetable mix (eggplant, zucchini, pumpkin, jilo, collard greens, etc.).

- Dinner: chicken skin with spinach and skin with white sauce.

Thursday

- Breakfast: Low carb panini with ham and cheese.
- Lunch: Horse steak with tomato and onion salad.
- Dinner: Ketogenic oven omelette with steamed broccoli.

Friday

- Breakfast: Bacon and Eggs.
- Lunch: Low-carb chicken and braised cabbage.
- Dinner: Pork chops with vegetables.

Saturday

- Breakfast: Low carbohydrate coconut mug muffin.
- Lunch: Mix the steamed vegetables with the ham and butter.
- Dinner: Low carb stuffed pizza of your choice.

Sunday

- Breakfast: Low-carb bread with eggs and cheese (click here for more carbohydrate breakfast ideas).

- Lunch: Barbecue (entitled to all meats, but stay away from garlic bread).
- Dinner: Zucchini Pasta with Bolognese Sauce.

Observations in the 7-day Ketogenic Diet Sample Menu

Remember to include too many low carbohydrate vegetables in your diet.After all, if your goal is to get less than 50 grams of carbs a day, there is room for a lot of vegetables in your diet - even if it's a low carbohydrate diet like a ketogenic diet.

Remember that vegetables, especially those high in fiber and low in starch, are the basis of a ketogenic diet.The goal is not to tell you exactly what to eat at each meal, but to provide ideas for tasty low-carb dishes and combinations between them.Based on this, you can always include or remove foods, depending on their availability, dietary restrictions and personal tastes.For example, if you are a vegetarian and want to follow a low carbohydrate diet, you can replace meat options with eggs, cheese or another source of protein.

04

KETONE FREQUENTLY ASKED QUESTIONS: KETOGENIC DIET FREQUENTLY ASKED QUESTIONS

01) Can I make garbage day in the ketogenic diet?

As we explained in the text about garbage day, it helps prevent weight loss from stagnating because carbohydrate intake (the basis of garbage day) helps raise the levels of some hormones essential for weight loss.

(Although reducing hormone T3 does not seem harmful on a ketogenic diet.)

Therefore, any carbohydrate feedback may be important to maintain a good level of these hormones. Therefore, we believe that it can be inserted into the ketogenic diet, but preferably only after your body has been adapted (about 4-5 weeks after starting the diet), and provided you have no clinical condition that can worsen with Carbohydrate intake.Remembering that in addition to the hormonal benefit, garbage day can also have great psychological benefit, making it more adherent to the diet. To make your life more enjoyable, you can do it. Health is a long term process, not just a focus on "weight loss now".

02) Can I eat cold cuts on this diet?

Although they are processed foods with a large amount of preservatives, looking only with regard to carbohydrates, we can say that sausages in general have low carbohydrate, because they have little or no carbohydrate in its composition, adapting to the ketogenic diet.Also, cheeses are usually released. In this case, prioritize high-fat, low-carbohydrate yellow cheeses.

03) How many meals should I eat during the day?

With the introduction of a low carbohydrate diet, and therefore more focused on protein and fat, it is natural for your appetite to gradually subside.Eat as many meals as you like, always feel satiated, remembering that the most important thing is not to get hungry to the point of "pinching" the absurd.But most importantly, you don't have to worry about breaks - forget the "eat every 3 hours" lie.

04) I'm vegetarian, can I do the ketogenic diet too? How should I proceed?

Yes you can.Therefore, to get all the necessary macronutrients from food alone, it would be interesting to focus on getting your daily protein and fat intake - just eggs and cheese can help you.

05) Do I need to be aware of the amount of fat ingested?

No. As we explained in the article on ketosis, you are unlikely to eat too much fat.On the other hand, we don't find it necessary to add butter and coconut oil to everything you see ahead.Even excess and lack of fat characterize common mistakes made by low-carb starters.Focus on eating the natural fat from foods (including bacon and egg yolk), you can fry with butter smoothly, beat in olive oil.

06) What can I eat for breakfast?

This is an excellent question, because breakfast with the ketogenic diet is a difficulty for many people.Sure, you can eat eggs and bacon - but not many people eat exactly that every day.And with that in mind, we have prepared a collection of low-carb breakfast cookbooks - which is perfect for the Ketone Diet.

07) Is milk a permitted food in the ketone diet?

As a rule, we can say no for two main reasons.First, because milk is a major cause of food allergies, it is not well tolerated by most people.Second, because it is a carbohydrate-rich food (lactose), it certainly doesn't go with ketosis.

08) Does the ketogenic diet also decrease lean mass or just fat?

In most diets, it is virtually impossible to lose just fat - that is, the most common is that a little lean mass and water is also lost.That said, there are measures to minimize the loss of lean mass in a diet.For example, you can practice a sport like bodybuilding, which helps preserve muscle mass and maintain good protein intake.

Finally, there is still the rarest case of people with enough weight to lose who are new to the sport.In this case, fat loss and mass gain can occur simultaneously!

Therefore, the goal is not to "find a diet that only loses fat" - but to minimize the loss of lean mass while burning fat.

09) I always thought fruits fit all diets, but should I cut them to lose weight with the ketogenic diet?

Fruits alone are not bad, their big problem is related to the high carbohydrates that most fruits have.On the other hand, there are some fruits with less sugar that can be consumed in the Keto diet, such as avocado, coconut and red fruits (eg strawberry and blueberry).

10) Oat bran is recommended in the Dukan diet, so can it also be used in the ketone diet?

The answer is no: oatmeal is a carbohydrate-rich food and should therefore be avoided or at most consumed in very low amounts, as in a recipe, for example.

11) And flaxseed meal, wheat, amaranth, quinoa ...?

In general, bran has a considerable amount of carbohydrate - despite many fibers - and consuming it without moderation can end up harming your ketosis.Therefore, the recommendation is always to examine the nutritional information and ensure that you do not consume too many carbohydrates, causing you to overflow the proportion considered ideal for the ketogenic diet.Not to mention that wheat can cause other health damage - far beyond carbohydrates.On the other hand, if you have read this far and have had this doubt, you may not have fully understood what the ketogenic diet is all about.And that's fine: It really must be a new world for you, full of different concepts from those you were used to hearing.Therefore, we recommend that you access our list and menu of free foods for the ketogenic diet.

And finally, if you want to delve deeper into and understand the daily life of this lifestyle, we invite you to discover our premium material by clicking here.

12) Are coffee and tea allowed on the ketone diet?

Yes, they are very welcome as long as they are not sweetened.Remembering that too much caffeine can be harmful to health, it is not recommended to exceed the limit of 4 cups of strong coffee a day.

13) Are beans, lentils and vegetables generally released in the ketone diet?

In the ketogenic diet, beans, lentils and other legumes are not consumed.

The main reason is associated with the presence of large amounts of carbohydrates (in addition to antinutrients) in these foods.If you like to eat these foods, I suggest you try to learn more about the Slow Carb diet.

14) I have reached a certain weight and I cannot get out of it, how should I proceed?

We talked about four essential tips for getting off the plateau on a low-carb diet in another text (we even recorded a video talking about it)

15) Can cereal bars, whole grain breads and cookies, breakfast cereals and tapioca gum be included in this diet?

Definitely, these foods are not released because they are high in carbohydrates that would certainly hinder your weight loss and insulin regulation process.Make no mistake, in most cases "whole" foods are almost as bad for your health and weight loss as their traditional versions.We even wrote a full post to demystify the healthy aura that tapioca has recently gained.

16) Are the ketogenic diet and the "protein diet" the same thing?

No they are not.

In fact, the term "protein diet" does not even refer to a specific diet as it is a very generic term. Generally speaking, people refer to some type of low carbohydrate diet when using this term, or even to the Dukan diet.

However, we cannot say that the ketone diet is a "protein diet" because in the ketogenic diet the amount of protein should be moderate and the most abundant macronutrient is fat.

17) Can you make a ketogenic diet with hypothyroidism or Hashimoto's disease?

In principle yes. The hypothyroidism that conditions are the foods that can be taken, but it does not condition the fact that it is a diet high in fat and low in carbohydrates. The ketogenic diet can be done with hypothyroidism but adapting it to the particular needs of the disease and the person, personalizing the recommendations.

18) How to know if the state of ketosis is optimal?

The most reliable and objective is to measure the concentration of ketone bodies in the blood, and for this, there are different devices. Blood measurement is more expensive, but also more accurate. These devices measure the blood concentration of ketone bodies and glucose with a drop of blood from the finger. We use a fairly reliable brand, Precision Xtra.

There are also test strips to measure ketone bodies in urine, a simpler and cheaper method, but less accurate.

19) How long is it advisable to do a ketogenic diet, a few months or as a long-term habit?

The strict ketogenic diet that is very high in fat and very low in carbohydrates and starches, is a therapeutic tool, it is like a medical treatment. This diet as such has a prescription time and must be very controlled, in fact, the ketogenic diet for severe cases of epilepsy or brain tumors, for example, is done in hospitals and is monitored daily.

When we make a ketogenic diet to improve our quality of life, our global health and lead a ketogenic lifestyle, the idea is to enter and exit. Make a tighter ketogenic diet around 4 weeks, and then make a window of a week in which we increase the intake of healthy carbohydrates. No industrial pastries, croissants, cookies, and sugars, etc. We would introduce carbohydrates, for example, from rice, from whole-grain cereals of organic production, a greater amount of fruit or legumes, vegetables with a higher starch load, such as green beans for example. That way we would do four-week strict keto cycles and one week with higher carbohydrate intake. In this way, the metabolic flexibility of which we have talked so much is gained, being healthier in the long term.

There are those who prefer not to do a ketogenic diet on a regular basis and two or three times a year to do a cycle in ketosis. This option can also be interesting.

In this sense, there is a range of possibilities. There are people who are more frequently in keto and go out from time to time and people who are barely there and enter a couple of times a year.

There are many intermediate options, but always adapting it to the needs of each one. In a serious disease where the objective of the ketogenic diet is to achieve a state of ketosis that will be therapeutic, as a curative treatment, because in that case, you have to be more strict; But if what you want is a lifestyle, or you want to get an extra sports or intellectual performance, then you can afford more flexibility.

The message that has to be clear is that a continuous ketogenic diet is not healthy, it is not recommended, and the healthy thing is to get in and out.

20) Can the ketogenic diet be done if the meat is not consumed?

Yes, you can, but in a ketogenic diet you have to resort to proteins of good quality and high biological value, and these are fundamental of animal origin. Therefore if the meat is not consumed, but if eggs and fish, in principle there is no problem. Now, if you do not eat meat or products of animal origin, it will be more complicated, because protein intake will come from legumes, for example, and legumes have a lot of starch. In the latter case, it will be much harder to get.

21) Can a flaxseed or chia seed be used in a ketogenic diet? How and in what quantity can it be used? And what foods do they combine with?

Yes, they can be used in different ways. Flaxseed or flax and chia seeds go very well for constipation problems. They can be taken as if it were a supplement, a food-medicine. They are soaked overnight, and the next morning, on an empty stomach, after drinking water and hydrating you can take a spoonful of these softened and anti-nutrient free seeds. You can also grind the chia and throw it, for example, into yogurt or salad.

22) Is the ketogenic diet related to the blood type based diet?

Yes and no. Everything is related.

No, because the ketogenic diet that defines is the proportion of nutrients, it is a diet very high in fat, very low in carbohydrates, moderate in protein and looking for a metabolic state of ketosis. But it is advisable to enrich the ketogenic diet taking into account the blood group because this way we customize the diet for each one.

Therefore yes, and it would be a ketogenic diet adapted to each person in group 0, A, B or AB. The most interesting thing is to make nutritional recommendations taking into account all the factors that influence our health. There are those who use it separately, to make a ketogenic diet, or diet according to the blood group, or diet to improve the intestine or diet for the skin ... The most natural, healthiest and most beneficial is to fuse all these aspects and find the best for each.

23) Can coffee be sweetened with organic honey in the ketogenic diet or is ketosis slowed?

Honey has a high glycemic index, so even if it is a small amount of honey, it leaves ketosis. To benefit from the dozens of beneficial properties that honey has it would have to be very good honey, not a distilled honey to which sugar is then added. In any case, it should be a very very small amount and in the ketogenic diet honey is super restricted, therefore it is not recommended.

24) How is organic chicken recognized? How is organic beef recognized?

Before buying the meat it is difficult to recognize it because we can only be guided by color, for example in red meat the color will be more intense, by consistency and by certification looking for quality seals that recognize organic production.

After buying meat is necessary to have the capacity to observe, body awareness and notice what we put in our mouths. We will look at the smell, color, consistency, and taste. In taste buds, it is noted for the taste and texture. But in order to have wise, aligned and intelligent taste buds, it is necessary to have a healthy diet, since when we eat processed foods in our diet, such as sugars, trans fats or foods with flavor enhancers such as monosodium glutamate, hypertrophy of our taste buds and we stop perceiving the most subtle flavors. For this reason, there are people who, when they go from a diet with processed foods and with the presence of all these substances, to a healthy diet, say that the food tastes like nothing. It's not that the food is tasteless,

In geographical areas with a lot of livestock tradition, when organic meat is eaten, the taste reminds us of the meat we ate when we were little, this is much better distinguished by older people. In recent years, the development and use of additives and substances that are added in the production of food have increased and that changes the taste, so it is a good indication of good quality meat when it has that aged flavor.

25) Can you make a ketogenic diet with triglycerides and high cholesterol?

This is one of the most discussed aspects of a ketogenic diet. For many people and professionals, the drawback of the ketogenic diet is the intake of high amounts of fats.The elevation of blood fats, cholesterol, and triglycerides, is closely related to the intake of sugars, carbohydrates and refined flours. This is a fundamental issue that is not usually discussed. If we want to control blood cholesterol and triglyceride levels, the first thing to remove from the diet is those foods or substances.When we make a ketogenic diet there is a mobilization of fats. When we are in ketosis, or when fasting we drink a tea or ketogenic coffee, fat burning is activated, there is a mobilization of fat deposits and transiently there may be a rise in blood fats.

The great manager of the body of fats in the liver. If the liver becomes saturated because it has to digest and process many fats, an elevation of cholesterol and triglycerides in the blood can be favored. That is why it is very important to do those cycles of entry and exit of the ketogenic diet and give the liver a break. To help the liver it is very important that a ketogenic diet includes fresh foods such as salads, lettuce, canons, arugula, and all green leafy vegetables, as they help the liver to detoxify and fulfill its functions.

Finally, it is very important to keep in mind that when there are high levels of blood fat, you have to have good control of blood sugar. If the levels are very high, you have to be very careful, but when we are talking about high levels of blood fat, but within a reasonable range, it is very important to control blood sugar, sugar, because that is what makes fat Be harmful. What makes the cholesterol sticky, adheres to the arterial walls and favors the development of atherosclerosis, thrombosis or embolisms, is that there is an inflammatory and glycosylation state, of the sum of sugar residues in these molecules, which makes it I hit the different structures .

26) Can the ketogenic diet be done without a gallbladder?

The gallbladder is a small organ, like a balloon when deflated, that does not fulfill a great function, said from this corseted structure of medicine that gives value to the large organs, to the noble organs; and if it gives any problem it can be removed. The function of the gallbladder is the storage and digestion of fats, the latter function that shares with the liver, bone that we do not lose that function to lose the gallbladder. But the truth is that people who have their gallbladder removed, have a number of problems with digestion and assimilation of nutrients, and with many more fats. That is why it will be very difficult to make a ketogenic diet without a gallbladder, at least until it has adapted. The agency has to find again its tools to process these foods in general and fats in particular. It is curious that this "balloon", that organ so insignificant and so discreet, has a very important role in these processes.

27) Can you follow a ketogenic diet and fast if you have Gilbert's syndrome?

Gilbert's syndrome is a liver involvement in which the liver does not process bilirubin properly. The disease is hereditary and has a characteristic feature that is that the person who suffers it turns yellow when he is very fatigued or when he makes physical or intellectual overexertion. In this case, it happens as in the previous case, we have a liver again with some difficulty to do its job and its metabolism. Therefore, it should be seen in each person, not in the Gilbert, but in that person who has a Gilbert syndrome, specifically. It will be more difficult and the capacity of each person will have to be assessed.

28) How is protein converted to glucose?

Basically, because the protein contains D-ribose. Ribose is a component of nucleic acids, it is a component of meat, it is a pentose, that is, a type of sugar. In the metabolism of meat and this ribose, when it is decomposing into its fundamental elements, it ends up fragmenting into glucose units. That is why if there is an excess of meat we end up having a higher blood glucose elevation. The sugar content in the meat is seen when cooking and leaving that kind of brown candy, that is the sugar in the meat.

29) Does the ketogenic diet improve inflammation in people with Sibo?

And it is. Sibo is a bacterial overgrowth syndrome at the intestinal level. Overgrowth and mobilization, since the bacterial population of one area of the intestine, colonizes another area of the intestine generating gas problems, discomfort, abdominal pain and intestinal rhythm disorder in addition to all those associated with poor health of the intestinal flora , of the microbiota. Therefore a ketogenic diet can help because it reduces the level of global inflammation in the body, but above all, the imbalance of the intestinal flora should be a priority in the treatment. It would be necessary to begin by solving and balancing the problem of intestinal flora.

30) Can you fast by drinking zero soda or eating sugarless candy?

It is not recommended. Some people recommend the use of artificial sweeteners in ketogenic diets, but we do not recommend it. We do not recommend it for health since they are chemical products that take their toll and of which various associated health problems have been described, but also because it favors the accordion effect.

A chemical sweetener, and "sugar-free" candies carry them, has such a strong sweetening power that our body responds as if we had ingested a large amount of sugar. At that time a peak of hyperglycemia occurs and then a fall, that already alters us and also favors the appearance of a pro-inflammatory state and different health problems that we have already talked about in this book.

The accordion effect occurs in many slimming diets and many people who lose weight and then recover it, also recovering more of the weight they had at first. This is why we do not recommend it.

The best thing in a fast is to take nothing, not to take any solid food, you just have to hydrate. Some people defend dry fasting, but I think it is not convenient because we have to be well hydrated since our intestine suffers from dehydration or underdehydration. In addition to favoring in our body the elimination of toxins through the urine during this period of cleaning that hydration is necessary. If you want to sweeten or add a touch of flavor to the water you can add a little lemon.

31) How many times a week can we eat fat? How much fat can we eat a day?

You can and should eat good quality fat every day.

If that fat is included in the meat, for example in a roast, then a lot of fat would be eaten, but also a lot of protein, so it would come out of ketosis.

The amount of daily fat depends on each person, the weight of each person or the desired weight. We have a book on the ketogenic diet that also includes 80 recipes and in which we explain the formula to calculate the amounts of each nutrient in the diet.

32) Does the ketogenic diet need medical control?

A strict ketogenic diet requires strict monitoring. It is a diet where 80-90% of the caloric value of intakes is in the form of fats, is very fat and has to be controlled, so as is usually done in hospitals and with a therapeutic approach, it includes a close follow- up. Today it is difficult to incorporate a diet of this type in the public health system since many doctors pay or even encourage their patients to leave it because they believe that it is not good, often from ignorance.

There is a lack of knowledge, education and going out of old schemes learning and analyzing studies. The ketogenic diet is about to turn 100 and there is a lot of information and research that is still going on.

33) Why do I have trouble sleeping on a ketogenic diet? What can I do to sleep better?

Without knowing the specific case, it is difficult to know what to do, but as a general recommendation, it is necessary to improve sleep hygiene. Here you have a complete article on how to improve the quality of sleep. It is also advisable to adjust the biological clock, noting a positive response of the organism when we advance the schedules. But it is not only about advancing dinner to have digested before going to bed, but also when we go to bed that it shows a lot even in weight control. It has been seen that in people who want to lose weight, or even in thin people who have a lot of difficulty gaining weight, the response improves when the clock is adjusted and adapts to the biological clock.

34) Is fat bad for the heart, arteries, and brain?

It is bad depending on the type of fat and the state of glycosylation or adhesion of sugar-derived particles in these molecules.

35) Can ketosis be vegetarian or vegan?

Vegetarian people have very complicated entering ketosis, and vegans even more because they do not take any animal products.

On the other hand, there is another important issue and that is that many vegetarian or vegan people take tofu, soy derivatives and among others, we are not in favor of taking soy derivatives as a source of protein.

However, if they are beneficial as derivatives of soy, fermented, miso and Tamari because they provide mainly probiotics, microorganisms that are very beneficial for intestinal flora apart from other interesting properties. For example, miso has shown a protective capacity against radiotherapy, for example. In people who are going to undergo radiotherapy for cancer, it is very interesting to include miso in the diet, for example, to drink a miso soup, add a little miso to the mash or cream of vegetables.

Out of these soy derivatives, the rest is not recommended. Because tofu, I'm milk or I'm drink, I'm yogurt, I'm sausages, I'm burgers, all-white derivatives of I'm are indigestible. Each person is different, but in general, they are indigestible and heavy because they are raw foods, which are not digested and intestinal work is more expensive. They are also allergens, please the response of our immune system and that favors the development of allergies, asthma, and dermatitis among others. For example, if a child who has asthma is removed from cow's milk as phenomenal, but if it is replaced by soy milk, his problem will not be solved much.

Finally, it is necessary to know, although it is not entirely clear, that the majority of soy that is consumed today is transgenic and it is not clear what the effect on the health of transgenic foods is.

36) What animal fats are of good quality?

First of all, they are from wild animals that have lived in a natural state or from animals cared for in an organic production system.

Of terrestrial origin the fat of the animals, the fat that is under the skin or the fat included in the muscular fascicles of different animals. If it can be hunting or animals that have been in the bush, or in the field in freedom, and if not those of organic production. This is a very important aspect because the fat concentrates the toxins, and if we take fat from animals that have been under a lot of stress or have eaten contaminated food or grass contaminated with herbicides and pesticides, we will take those toxins that are concentrated in the meat and in the fat. Eating that fat will bring us the benefits of fat and the inconvenience of all those toxins. Even of the endogenous toxins, the ones we manufacture, which is what happens, for example, in very stressed animals. The animals that live in housing, in large industrial buildings overcrowded and suffering, they release adrenaline, and that adrenaline is a toxin for them and for us. The liver metabolizes it, but in turn, it permeates the tissues. For all this, meat and fish of good quality are recommended.

From the sea, bluefish is recommended, which is very rich in essential fatty acids omega 3 and omega 6. Ideally, it should be wild, cold water and small or medium size to avoid heavy metal accumulation in large fish like the shark, the bluefin tuna, the swordfish since a large fish has been bioaccumulating for many years. It is better to consume small fish such as sardines, anchovies, mackerel, etc.

37) Is it safe to make a ketogenic diet during pregnancy?

The most important thing during pregnancy is that no drastic changes are made in the diet. Changes and preparations have to be made before pregnancy. There are critics of this diet that say that during pregnancy a ketogenic diet cannot be followed because the fetus is nourished and needs high levels of maternal glycemia feeding primarily on carbohydrates.

In the first place it is very important to adapt that woman to a ketogenic diet, she must have that metabolic flexibility of which we speak as well as a stable energy level and a healthy metabolic level with that alternation of entry and exit cycles accompanied by elevations in your intake of carbohydrates, vegetables, legumes, rice, etc. And in the case of being pregnant, it should be more frequent to maintain slightly higher blood sugar levels and lower ketosis.

38) Can you eat the fruit in the ketogenic diet?

In the ketogenic diet, the consumption of fruit is very restricted because, due to the sugar supply, it causes us to get out of ketosis. Therefore the fruit is very restricted to a small amount and low glycemic index, mainly fruits of the forest, blueberries, and raspberries. It is one of the disadvantages of the ketogenic diet, and that is why you can take advantage of those moments of flexibility to eat a little more fruit. The fruit does not contribute anything that other vegetables do not contribute, so you have to take the vitamins, minerals, and fiber of vegetables and vegetables. That is where we have to make all the emphasis and also that they are in good quantity to help the liver in its work of metabolizing fats.

39) Is fruit fructose good or bad for your health?

Fruit sugar or fructose is better than sugar in general. It is a sugar that we handle better, that has a slower metabolism and that does not give those peaks of hyperglycemia. Therefore the sugar of the fruit is better than that of a sweet for example. In addition to being a sweet food, it is accompanied by vitamins, minerals, and fiber, all of them very important nutrients for us.

The problem with fruit is that we eat it all year long. Our ancestors drank fruit at very specific moments, mainly at the end of the summer, which was when the fruits had matured by gathering them. This helped to increase their fat stores because the increase in sugar favored fat storage, and accumulating that extra energy as fat they protected themselves against the inclemency of the winter and the shortage of food. But they also dried the fruit to eat it as fruit steps, such as dates, prunes, figs steps, etc. This is very important and there is a clear difference between drinking fruit all year round and drinking it at a specific time.

On the other hand, what kind of fruits did our ancestors eat? Well, mainly fences and small fruits of the forest with a lower glycemic index.

Finally, we must talk about how fruits have evolved, hybrids have become and now we eat foods that are new in evolution. We adapt very quickly, but metabolically speaking we have an enzymatic system that is breaking and taking advantage of food and dating from the Paleolithic. We are trying to digest and absorb new foods well, such as nectarines and tangerines that are the result of hybridization, with an old metabolic system. For example, mandarins are more and more and more sweet hybrids, that's why today's mandarin is nothing like the tangerine of two centuries ago.

40) Does eating two eggs a day increase cholesterol?

Studies that have been done with the intake of eggs and the assessment of cholesterol levels have not shown that the consumption of eggs increases blood cholesterol.

41) Why is butter good and milk is bad?

The quality of the food itself and the origin of the animal must be studied.

In general, milk and cow products give us problems, in general, we tolerate goat and sheep milk better. There are others that can also be taken as buffalo in the mozzarella.

On the other hand, the quality of the food is very important. It is very different the quality and the impact that our milk, in general, has on our health that comes from an animal that has lived in freedom, or that has been cared for in an organic production system, that has eaten a good grass, etc. an example, because it is a food rich in omega 3. It seems to us that foods of animal origin do not have essential fatty acids omega 3, but this is not the case, the milk of a cow of organic production that eats grass, if it is rich in omega 3 and the fats derived from these dairy products, such as butter, even richer.

Another important aspect is the person who consumes these foods. I advise against them in general because they are associated with many health problems such as asthma, dermatitis, digestive problems, mood problems, depression, anxiety, cancer, some of them very seriously. But if the person, in general, has an optimal level of health and also an innate and adequate tolerance to these foods can consume them.

As for butter, the most important thing is that it is easier to digest. The main drawback of dairy products is that we cannot digest them well and that creates problems at the intestinal level leading to other aspects of health. This is partly because butter is fundamentally fat, it has neither the lactose that is sugar nor the casein that are milk proteins, and both are the factors involved in most of the problems derived from dairy consumption.

Butter is fundamentally fat, just over 80% is fat, 18% is water, a small percentage are mineral salts and 0.06% carbohydrates. It is, therefore, food that we metabolize much better and this is an important aspect. That is why milk does not butter itself, but with all these nuances and always butter of organic origin and preferably grass.

42) How to avoid the rebound effect when leaving ketosis?

The most important thing is that the ketogenic diet takes you to a ketogenic lifestyle, eat with that flexibility ketogenic-type and promptly leave or a more flexible type where we promptly enter ketosis; and accompany it with intermittent fasting and physical activity. Both very important in the ketogenic diet.

43) How is the ketogenic diet different from the Atkins diet?

The ketogenic diet is a diet high in fat, very low in carbohydrates, especially in starches and moderate in proteins, which wants to mimic the metabolic state of fasting with an operation based on ketone bodies as fuel. The Atkins is a diet rich in protein, and the ketogenic diet is a moderate protein diet because a high amount of protein takes us out of the state of ketosis since glucose units are generated in its metabolism.

05

FOODS IN THE KETOGENIC DIET

Do you have problems choosing food for a ketogenic diet?

Do you have trouble deciding which foods to include and which ones to avoid?

Choosing foods well for a ketogenic diet makes the difference between losing fat or gaining it.If your menu consists only of keto foods you will easily enter ketosis and start losing fat at an accelerated rate.On the other hand, if you eat what you don't touch, you will get out of ketosis and your body will accumulate the extra fat you are eating.To know the best foods for the ketogenic diet it is necessary to know the macronutrient composition of each food.

LOW CARB FRUITS

As a general rule in the ketogenic diet, the consumption of fruit must be limited.

The fruit is very rich in carbohydrates, especially short-chain carbohydrates, which are absorbed very quickly, and if you eat too much fruit you will leave ketosis almost immediately.Remember that to follow the ketogenic diet you can not exceed the consumption of 30 grams daily of carbohydrates.A single banana already contains 27 grams of carbohydrates, an apple 18 and an orange 15!So fruits, in general, are food for a ketogenic diet.But, if you do not want to give up the fruit completely, we recommend that you eat berries (or berries) especially as they contain the lowest levels of carbohydrates and coconut in moderation, which is high in fat.If you are able to resist the temptation you can also consume small amounts of cherries, strawberries, plums or a small piece of any other fruit, but we do not recommend it since easily a bite will become two or three and without realizing it you will have eaten Too much fruitTo get the micronutrients that the fruit gives you we recommend you eat a lot of vegetables.

Below, you will find a list of the low-carb fruits most suitable for the ketogenic diet along with the number of carbohydrates per 100 grams of these ingredients:

fruit Carbs in 100g

Avocado   2 grams

Raspberries 5 grams

Blackberries	5.7 grams
Strawberries	6 grams
Blueberries	6.1 grams
Cantaloupe	6.8 grams
Plums	7.5 grams
Watermelon	7.5 grams
Peach (or peach)	8.6 grams
Oranges and tangerines (or clementines)	9.3 grams
Cherries	10 grams
Kiwis	10.6 grams
Coconut (33.5 grams of fat)	15.2grams

VEGETABLES FOR A KETOGENIC DIET

Vegetables are the keto foods that will become your allies and that you have to eat in large quantities while you are ketosis.Not only will they provide you with essential micronutrients, but they will also be the source of fiber that you will need in a high-fat diet.It is important that the vegetables are seasonal and, where possible, organic farming since they are richer in micronutrients than greenhouse vegetables.

There is an easy rule to know what vegetables to eat:

- The vegetables you have to eat the most are the leaves or flowers
- Second, the fruits (beware! Fruits, not fruits)
- The least recommended tubers and bulbs

LEAF OR FLOWER VEGETABLES

These vegetables are the best foods for a ketogenic diet. You can eat as many as you want, they are low carb vegetables!

The only exception on this list is Kale, which although very nutritious, cannot be eaten in large quantities since it is rich in carbohydrates. These keto foods will fill the color plate and provide you with micronutrients and fiber.

Here is a list of vegetables with the number of carbohydrates they contain so you can choose your ketogenic diet foods:

Leaf or flower vegetables	Carbs in 100g
Spinach	3 grams
Canons	1 gram
Lettuce	2 grams
Chard	2 grams
Broccoli	2 grams
Cauliflower	3 grams

Endives	3 grams
Watercress	3 grams
Cabbage (or cabbage)	3 grams
Celery	3 grams
Arugula	4 grams
Kale	4 grams
Brussels sprouts	5 grams
Kale	8 grams

FRUIT VEGETABLES

These vegetables should be qualified as fruits, but culturally they have been differentiated from the sweetest fruits. They have a little more carbohydrates than leafy vegetables but their levels are low enough to be part of our food for a ketogenic diet.

Fruit vegetable	Carbs in 100g
Avocado	2 grams
Zucchini	3 grams
Green pepper	3 grams
Red pepper	4 grams

Cucumber	4 grams
Tomato	4 grams
Yellow pepper	5 grams
pumpkin	5.6 grams
Eggplant	6 grams

TUBERS IN THE KETOGENIC DIET

Within this category are the vegetables that grow underground. They are vegetables with higher levels of carbohydrates and therefore are not the best foods for a ketogenic diet and we will have to limit their presence in our ketogenic menu. The only exception is radishes.

Tuber	Carbs in 100g
Radish	3 grams
Carrot	7 grams
Onion	7 grams
Beet	7 grams
Turnip	7 grams
Swede	7 grams
Parsnip	13 grams

Potato (or potato)   15 grams

Sweet potato (or sweet potato)   17 grams

Garlic   24.3 grams

How can you observe there are some vegetables such as potatoes or sweet potatoes that are better to avoid completely since they will easily make you exceed the limit of 30 grams of carbohydrates daily.If you do not want to be weighing vegetables all day we suggest you stick to eating vegetables with less than 5 grams of carbohydrates / 100 grams of vegetables.You can eat as much as you want of these vegetables since you can hardly exceed the limits (you would have to eat 3 Kg of spinach a day to reach the limit!).

Avocado is itself a special category, its high-fat content makes it a great food keto. We recommend that you incorporate it into your 100% diet. A single avocado will give you 29 grams of healthy fat.

NUTS IN THE KETOGENIC DIET

Nuts, apart from being delicious, can be good foods for a ketogenic diet.They are very fatty foods and will help you diversify your ketogenic menu.

But not everything goes with nuts!

- The biggest risk they have is that being so appetizing and having such a high caloric load it is easy to end up overeating.

- The second problem is that some of them contain enough carbohydrates and if they are not eaten in moderation they can cause us to get out of ketosis.
- The third risk is that, like all seeds, they contain anti-nutrients that can generate an inflammatory response in our digestive system.

Avoiding these 3 risks is simple, you just have to follow these 3 rules:

- Only eat nuts low in carbohydrates such as pecans or macadamias and avoid especially cashews and pistachios
- Do not abuse them or eat roasted or salted nuts.
- Eat them raw and after soaking them overnight to eliminate toxins

In this comprehensive guide, you will find all the information you need about nuts.

Below, you will find a list of the most important nuts with their amounts of fat and carbohydrates per 100gr of this ingredient that you can incorporate into your ketogenic diet foods.

Dried fruit	Carbs / 100g	Fat / 100g
Macadamia nuts	5 grams	77 grams
Pecan Nuts	4 grams	72 grams
Walnuts	7 grams	66 grams
Pinions	9 grams	61 grams

Hazelnuts	7 grams	61 grams
Almonds	4 grams	50 grams
Cashew nuts	25 grams	46 grams
Peanut or peanut	7.9 grams	46 grams
Pistachios	18 grams	45 grams
Sunflower seeds	43 grams	20 grams
Pumpkin Pipes	49.1 grams	10.7grams

Attention, peanuts (or peanuts) are not really a dried fruit, they are a legume. We have included them here because they are commonly confused. We recommend you avoid them.

A final reminder: avoid salted and fried nuts.

Salt generates a sensation of immediate pleasure and induces us to eat more than we need. The same goes for the fat in fried nuts, with the aggravating fact that fried foods contain carcinogenic compounds that are not good for our health.

LEGUMES AND CEREALS IN THE KETOGENIC DIET

This is the easiest list to make: completely avoid eating legumes and cereals as part of your food for a ketogenic diet.

The reasons are several:

- They are foods rich in carbohydrates and very poor in fat.

- They do not have any micronutrient that you cannot get with vegetables or meat, fish or eggs.

- They are rich in antinutrients (especially cereals).

Whether you follow a ketogenic diet menu, such as low carb or simply a healthy diet, our recommendation is that you avoid cereals to the maximum and minimize the consumption of legumes.

We want to highlight a cereal that you have to avoid especially: wheat.Its high gluten content makes it a bad choice in your diet you can read more information in this book.

MEAT, FISH AND OTHER SOURCES OF PROTEIN

In any healthy diet, you have to have a source of protein.Meat, fish, and eggs are therefore necessary for a ketogenic diet.But it is also important not to abuse.If you eat too much protein, your body will use the excess to generate glucose in a process called "gluconeogenesis." This is especially important at the beginning when you want to go into ketosis.

On the other hand, if you do not eat enough protein, your body will not be able to regenerate muscle efficiently and, during the ketogenic diet, in addition to losing fat, you will also lose muscle, something that does not suit you.

This is important if you combine the ketogenic diet with exercise.We recommend you do it, especially training with HIIT, as it will increase your metabolism and burn fat faster.

To know how much protein to eat we suggest this rule:

- If you are not an athlete, eat 1 gram of protein / Kg of body mass
- If you are an athlete, eat 2 grams of protein / Kg of body mass

To know how much protein is in each food look at the following table:

Food Protein / 100g

Meat	26 grams
Fish	25 grams
Seafood	24 grams
Eggs	13 grams (6g / egg)
Chicken	11 grams

Our recommendation is that you use eggs as the main source of protein. They are high in fat and more sustainable. Again, it is important that they be free-range chicken eggs and, if possible, grass (not eating cereals).You can know more about the consumption of eggs and their effect on cholesterol here.Fish and shellfish are also very good sources of protein, especially small fish such as sardine, which is a great source of omega 3, has a low ecological impact and little heavy metal accumulation.

SUPPLEMENT FOR THE KETOGENIC DIET

The ketogenic diet, if you follow this guide, does not require any supplementation, since you will get all the necessary micronutrients with the vegetables, meat, fish and eggs you will consume.But it is true that during the process of adaptation to the ketogenic diet some discomforts can arise that are easily solvable with the strategic consumption of supplementation.

We also have to keep in mind that many of the foods we consume today are poor in some minerals because of over-exploitation of the soil. The most pragmatic case is that of magnesium, of which a large part of the population has deficiencies.

In this keto guide, we will give you a complete guide on the supplementation to take.

- Omega 3: It is a basic component of your brain and you will only find it in sufficient quantities in bluefish or shellfish. It may be a good idea to supplement 1000 mg of DHA daily.
- Vitamin C: Stimulant of the use of ketones by neurons and to increase the manufacture of transporters in the blood-brain barrier.
- Magnesium: Consuming an adequate amount of magnesium will prevent muscle cramps and digestive

problems that sometimes arise when a person enters ketosis for the first time.

KETOGENIC DIET RECIPES

The keto or ketogenic diet is one that produces in our body a process called ketosis that can be very useful when burning fat and producing important metabolic changes. To achieve this, hydrates must be considerably restricted from there, which is a diet that requires limited control and time for its realization.

Recipes for breakfast or snack

Since in the keto diet it is not possible to go to cereals and derivatives or to bread, fruits or starchy vegetables, our breakfasts and snacks will change considerably.

Some recipes rich in protein and fat foods that we can prepare for these meals are:

- Cloud eggs: they are ideal for a quick breakfast with nothing but egg, although we can serve it with bacon as the recipe shows, or with seeds, nuts, avocado or simply with chicken breast or cooked turkey.
- Omelet: it is one of the most basic and easy options for our breakfasts. We can serve it alone or, accompany it with avocado or cheese if we want to add a different flavor.
- Eggs in a serrano ham casserole: it is another egg-based alternative that allows us to solve the first meal of the

day easily and with many proteins as well as satiating power.

- Avocados with baked eggs: ideal for protein, healthy fats and a variety of vitamins and minerals in our first meal of the day without resorting to foods rich in carbohydrates.

- Cloud bread or cloud bread: ideal for bread lovers who miss this food. It is easy to prepare and we can combine it with cheese, with ham, avocado, olive oil or as many ingredients as the keto diet allows us.

Recipes for lunch or dinner

To solve the main meals without resorting to cereals and derivatives, legumes or vegetables or fruits, we will use meat, fish, cheese, and eggs in different preparations:

- Cod omelet: very easy to make and packed with protein. It includes a minimum of vegetables that will not affect ketosis but we could also remove them from the recipe if necessary.

- Eggs stuffed with tuna: rich in healthy fats and proteins that satisfy this recipe is ideal for a simple dinner or as an appetizer or starter of a more complete menu.

- Greek salad pan: if necessary we can avoid the tomato and onion of the recipe, although the amount of hydrates per serving is too low to interfere with ketosis. That dish is ideal for an easy meal but very satiating and rich in good fats.

- Light tuna quiche: for lunch or dinner this quiche is very easy to make and is very attractive to the eye as well as to the palate. If we wish we can change the tuna for another fish without inconvenience.

- Baked chicken breasts with Morbier cheese: with many proteins that satisfy and extra calcium due to the recipe cheese, this dish is ideal for lunch or dinner.

- Poached eggs with gulas and prawns: for pecking or to serve as a colorful entree of a more complete menu to entertain guests this may be the ideal recipe that respects your keto diet.

- Roasted avocados with mozzarella: it is a very simple preparation that although we can use it for breakfast, it goes very well as an entree or for a light dinner.

- Baked salmon with nuts: a recipe filled with omega 3, ideal for satiating at lunch or dinner due to its richness in protein and fiber.

For the Ketogenic Diet, they have indicated a series of foods that are allowed and many others that are prohibited, giving them the freedom to personally choose their daily menu, however, we provide an example of how they can organize their meals. Remember that you will do it depending on the stage you are in.

Breakfast: Start the day with some good scrambled eggs with ham.

Mid-morning: You can make a lettuce salad with virgin olive oil.

Snack or Snack: A handful of nuts will satisfy your hunger.

Food: Make a roast chicken that you can accompany with avocado in the form of a salad, and for dessert a skimmed yogurt.

Dinner: You can use a grilled salmon, accompanied by baked vegetables and a piece of goat cheese.

Snack: take a good dietary jelly.

Fat Burner vs Sugar Burner: When you eat something that is high in carbohydrates (that delicious donut), your body will produce glucose and insulin.

Glucose is the easiest molecule for your body to convert and use as energy, so it is the source of energy preferred by your body.Insulin is produced to process glucose in your bloodstream by transporting it throughout your body.This sounds pretty efficient, right? The problem with this is that when glucose is used as a primary energy source, fats are not necessary for energy and are therefore stored.With an average person's diet, glucose is the main source of energy.

This initially does not seem to be a problem until you realize that the body cannot store so much glucose. This becomes a problem for you because the extra glucose is converted into fat that is then stored.Because your body uses glucose as its main source of energy, glucose that is converted to fat is not used.When your body runs out of glucose, it tells your brain that you need more, so you end up looking for a quick snack like a candy bar or some fries.

You can start to see how this cycle leads you to build a body that you really don't want.

So what is the alternative?

Become a fat burner instead of a sugar burner.

When you decrease your carbohydrate intake, the body begins to look for an alternative energy source and your body enters a metabolic state known as ketosis.

Ketosis is a natural process and it makes sense when you think about the human body. You have probably heard of the fact that you can spend weeks without food, but only a couple of days without water. The reason for this is ketosis. Most people, for better or worse, have enough fat stored in them to feed their body for a while. When your body is in a state of ketosis, it produces ketones. Ketones are produced by the breakdown of fat in the liver.

You might be thinking why the body does not constantly break down fats in the liver? Well, when your body produces insulin, insulin prevents fat cells from entering the bloodstream to remain stored in the body. When you reduce your carbohydrate intake, glucose levels, along with blood sugar levels, decrease, which in turn reduces insulin levels.

This allows fat cells to release the water they are storing (which is why a drop in water weight is first seen) and then fat cells are able to enter the bloodstream and go to the liver. This is the ultimate goal of the ketogenic diet. Ketosis is not entered into by starving the body. You enter ketosis by depriving your body of carbohydrates. When your body is producing optimal levels of ketones, you begin to notice many benefits of healing, weight loss, and physical and mental performance.

Total Carbs vs. Net Carbs

It is important to understand that not all carbohydrates are treated in the same way when looking at a nutrition label.

On the nutritional labels, you will total carbohydrates along with an additional breakdown of fiber and sugars.

In ketogenic diets, you are concerned about net carbohydrates that are total carbohydrates - Fiber = net carbohydrates.

Because fiber does not affect your blood sugar levels, it is considered a zero net carbohydrate.

Vegetables in a ketogenic diet

Vegetables are difficult on a ketogenic diet because we have been raised under the idea that vegetables are healthy and they are. However, almost all the vegetables you consume today contain carbohydrates.

Some more than others so it is important to understand those who have a safer number of net carbohydrates.

Amount of vegetables Net carbohydrates

Spinach (Raw) 1/2 Cup 0.1

Bok Choi 1/2 cup 0.2

Echuga (Roman) 1/2 cup 0.2

Cauliflower (steamed) 1/2 cup 0.9

Cabbage (raw green) 1/2 cup 1.1

Cauliflower (raw) 1/2 cup 1.4

Broccoli (Florets) 1/2 Cup 2

Kale 1/2 Cup 2

Kale (steamed) 1/2 cup 2.1

Green beans (steamed) 1/2 cup 2.9

Exercise on the ketogenic diet

The concern of people who exercise is that the ketogenic diet will affect your physical performance and although this is not true in the long term, in the short term you could experience a small fall.

Your body needs a little time to adapt.

The good news is that studies (in trained cyclists) have shown that those who follow the ketogenic diet did not find a compromise in their aerobic endurance or a loss of muscle mass.

06

LOW CARB AND HIGH-FAT DIETS

Carbohydrates make us fat, right? This common mistake comes from the claim that carbohydrates are bad for us because they are converted to glucose, causing the release of insulin, which helps the body store any excess energy in the form of fat. However, it is not only carbohydrates that stimulate the secretion of insulin, protein and high-fat food, but they also do too. In fact, too much energy from any nutritional source will lead to weight gain.

Over the years there have been many versions of the low carb and high-fat diet (the LCHF diet), eg Atkins, Dukan and the most recent, the ketogenic diet, but all have the same feeding model: a very low carbohydrate intake (approximately 20-50 g per day), high fat and a moderate protein intake. Diets normally involve the exclusion of grains, legumes, dairy products, refined sugar and most starchy fruits and vegetables. The carbohydrates in these diets come from non-starchy vegetables, nuts, and seeds. The LCHF diet defends the claim that diets can help you lose weight, control hunger and improve health. Some confirm that LCHF diets can be used as a cancer treatment.

Is there any science that supports these claims?

Research shows that, when carefully planned, the LCHF diet can be an effective treatment for people suffering from epilepsy and can help control type 2 diabetes. There is also evidence that very low carb diets can result in increased weight loss for people with obesity compared to low-fat diets. However, any weight loss that occurs is probably the result of the lack of calories created by the exclusion of energy-rich food and following an extremely low carbohydrate diet could be for many people a not so practical and long-lasting option term. In addition, many carbohydrates found in food, such as fruits, vegetables, and whole grains, contain important components for health, including vitamins, minerals and dietary fiber.

Although the use of the ketogenic diet (the LCHF diet) in cancer treatment has shown promising results, further research is necessary to better explain the effects. The limited number of studies and the differences in their designs and characteristics, which end up giving evidence of poor quality, make it very difficult to draw a firm, factual conclusion.

How do carbohydrates fit into a healthy diet?

The carbohydrates are a type of macronutrients found in most foods and are a very important part of our diets. They become glucose, which the body uses as a source of energy to maintain the functioning of muscles and organs. Various types of carbohydrates differ by chemical composition, digestion rate, and absorption:

Simple carbohydrates are made up of one or two sugar molecules and our body digests and absorb them quickly. The added sugar and sugar found in fruits or milk are examples of simple carbohydrates.

Complex/starchy carbohydrates are made up of a long chain of sugar and take longer to digest. Examples of complex carbohydrates include potatoes, legumes, and whole grains eg brown rice, barley, and oats.

Dietary fiber is the carbohydrate of plant origin that differs from simple or complex carbohydrates because it is not digested in the small intestine and, therefore, reaches the large intestine. Fiber helps keep our digestive system healthy and prevent constipation.

Foods rich in fiber, such as fruits or vegetables, whole wheat bread/pasta, nuts, and seeds can contribute to maintaining weight since they can give the feeling of fullness and satiety.

The European Food Safety Authority (EFSA) recommends a carbohydrate intake of between 45 and 60 percent of total energy intake for both adults and children and the World Health Organization (WHO) recommends that less than 10% of carbohydrate intake should come from free sugars. Eating a variety of foods that contain carbohydrates gives maximum nutritional benefit.

Research shows that unnecessarily eliminating a group of foods from the diet can lead to nutrient deficiency and create a negative relationship with food, which can cause, in extreme cases, an eating disorder. It is important to remember that balance, variety and portion control is the key.

DAIRY PRODUCTS THAT COULD RUIN YOUR KETOGENIC DIET

Many people who follow the ketogenic diet depend on cheese and other dairy products to get the amount of fat and protein needed, but not all dairy products are the same. This is what you should know.

- People who follow the ketogenic diet or Keto have to restrict their carbohydrates to less than 30 grams per day.
- It is important to evaluate the number of carbohydrates in each food to stay in ketosis or fat-burning mode.
- Some foods, such as milk or yogurt, can contain up to 24 grams of carbohydrates and can keep people from ketosis.

As anyone who follows a ketogenic diet already knows, the lifestyle requires a lot of diligence. Even having a banana could ruin your diet. The main objective of Keto is to use fat instead of carbohydrates for energy, a process known as ketosis. In general, people who do the Keto diet eat a lot of fat, a moderate amount of protein and only 20-30 grams of carbohydrates per day to maintain ketosis. That is, about half of a medium roll.

Some foods, such as bread, are known for their carbohydrates, so it is not surprising that you get out of the state of ketosis. But there are many foods that at the minimum could make your diet out of adjustment.

If you're trying to stay diligent with the Keto diet, check the nutritional information of these six amazing sources of carbohydrates.

1) Milk

Milk is a great source of protein and fat, but 1 cup of 2 percent milk contains 13 grams of carbohydrates. Since you are likely to eat other carbohydrate foods during the day, such as vegetables or nuts, that glass of milk can put you on the recommended 30 grams of carbohydrates per day.

2) Cottage cheese

Low in fat and high in protein, cottage cheese has long been a staple for many dieters. However, people who follow the Keto diet should be careful when eating cottage cheese in abundance. A single small cup of cottage cheese has approximately 8 grams of carbohydrates. Although it may be good to eat it only as an appetizer, be careful to combine it with other foods that have traces of carbohydrates, such as avocados and nuts.

3) Yogurt

The nut-covered yogurt may seem like a Keto snack without complications, but a 150-gram serving of plain yogurt has 12 grams of carbohydrates. If you opt for yogurt flavors, such as vanilla, the carbohydrate content doubles to 24 grams of carbohydrates per 170 gr. Your best option is to choose a simple Greek yogurt, which contains only five grams of carbohydrates per serving of 200 gr.

Why Does The Ketogenic Diet Work?

For many years, nutritionists have preached that in order to lose weight it was necessary to eat fewer calories.Their argument was that there is an energy balance in your body:

- If you eat more than you spend: you accumulate fat.
- If you eat less than you spend: you burn fat.

So to lose weight or burn more energy or eat less.

Your logic is overwhelming, right? but something fails .Apart from eating little is really torture, the practice does not correspond to the theory.Many of us have tried these types of diets and the result is that we either lose the weight we wanted or when we leave them we recover it again.The explanation is that the accumulation of fat in the body is not just a matter of energy balance, it is the result of a metabolic process that emerged from millions of years of evolution.

To understand what happens we have to review the evolution and basic biology:Human beings have lived millions of years in a world of scarcity.Until very recently, our ancestors suffered recurring famine.Therefore accumulating energy was necessary to survive.And how do we accumulate energy?

An adult has:

- Glycogen (carbohydrate) reserves that allow you to survive 1 or 2 days maximum.

- Reserves in the form of fat equivalent to more than 100,000 KCal or 50 days of survival.

CARBOHYDRATE METABOLISM

The carbohydrates we eat are processed within our body to their basic molecule, glucose. The absorption of glucose and its transport in the blood is very fast. This is good if we are going to use it at the moment, but bad if we don't need it.

Blood glucose levels are always maintained in a very narrow range of 72-145 mg / dl, or about 5 g total for an adult. Higher levels are toxic. When we eat carbohydrates the body perceives a rise in blood glucose and:

- Burn it immediately
- It releases the hormone insulin that tells the body that it has to store the excess glucose inside the cells, in the form of glycogen or fat.

When glucose reaches our cells, it "burns" very quickly through a process called glycolysis. This process has low energy efficiency.

Glycolysis can be done both without the presence of oxygen (anaerobic metabolism) and generates 2 or 3 ATPs / glucose (the energy currency of the cell), or in the presence of oxygen (aerobic metabolism) where a total of 32 ATPs is generated.

FAT METABOLISM - KETOSIS

Our body has the ability to use fatty acids (fats) as a source of energy through beta-oxidation of fats.Unlike glucose, fatty acids are absorbed more slowly and are more difficult to "burn." In fact, we need mitochondria to do it.

(Mitochondria are the power plants of our cells and the most surprising thing is that billions of years ago were bacteria that were installed inside another cell in a symbiosis relationship.)The transformation of fats into energy is called "beta-oxidation" and can only be done in aerobic conditions and is a much slower process than glycolysis.Fatty acids degrade up to 3 basic molecules: acetyl-Co-A that enters the citric acid cycle, NADH and FADH2.This process is so efficient that about 120 ATPs are obtained depending on the length of the fatty acid chain (remember that only 32 ATPs came out of glycolysis).

KETOSIS AND THE BRAIN

The brain consumes 20% of our body's energy.For a long time it was considered that fats were not a good "fuel" since they cannot be used by the brain as energy for two reasons:

- They cannot cross the blood-brain barrier.
- Some brain cells do not have mitochondria.
- By cons, the brain can consume glucose very well.

This is one of the most used reasons to recommend carbohydrates as the main source of energy.

Now we know that this is only half true. Even better food for the brain has been discovered: ketone bodies.

There is enough scientific evidence behind this statement:

- The ketone bodies are very effective in reaching the brain
- They have antioxidant and free radical reduction effects via Coenzyme Q regulation
- Increased concentrations of polyunsaturated fatty acids that have a neuroprotective effect
- Increase GABA neurotransmitter expression

Our body does not store ketone bodies, so our liver is prepared to produce them from fats. Beta-hydroxybutyrate represents up to 70% of the energy used by the brain and is produced only in the liver from fatty acids.

WHAT HAPPENS WHEN WE START GIVING CARBOHYDRATES CONSTANTLY TO OUR BODY?

Too many carbohydrates in our diet and eating too many times a day causes our body to adapt to using only glucose as a source of energy. As glucose stores are very limited and are consumed very quickly the body can only be obtained from outside. This generates addiction. Surely you will have heard about the addiction that causes sugar. Well, it is just this. The body depends on the glucose we eat for energy since it has "forgotten" how to use fats. Another more serious problem of eating too much sugar is that it induces too high levels of insulin in the blood, which in the worst-case generates resistance and ends in diabetes.

THE KETOGENIC DIET AND SPORTS PERFORMANCE

It has long been thought that elite athletes need to eat 4 or 5 times a day so as not to lose muscle mass and recover well from workouts.With the ketogenic diet and metabolism in ketosis this is no longer necessary.Fat metabolism is much more efficient. Therefore, by eating less we get more energy.

This implies that with just 2 meals a day we can get all the energy needed to perform and leave us time to be fasting that induces greater cell regeneration.

High concentrations of ketone bodies in the blood promotes greater DNA compaction that is more protected from oxidation damage. This affects the speed of recovery after exercising.

But ketone bodies don't work for everything.

When we enter anaerobic metabolism (sprints, HIITs ...), not enough oxygen reaches the cell. Then glucose enters into action with anaerobic metabolism.This change in metabolism does not have to worry you, it is very healthy that the body adapts to different energy needs

In summary: Training in ketosis gives us more energy, we recover faster and we need to eat less giving the body time to regenerate better, but always within the aerobic metabolism.

INFLAMMATION

Studies have shown that the levels of pro-inflammatory cytokines such as interleukin 1 beta, TNF alpha and interleukin 6 are reduced when we enter ketosis

KETOGENIC DIET AND CANCER

In many types of tumors, mitochondria degrade and therefore depend solely on glycogenesis to grow. This is called the Warburg effect. If we reduce glucose levels we can literally kill hunger cancer

MUSCLE MASS

There are several studies that have shown that ketogenic diets not only have a minor effect on the loss of muscle mass compared to other diets but also allow this mass to be maintained with lower protein intake. These cases can be anecdotal and it is not known what mechanism they follow.

LONGEVITY

Although little is known about the effect of ketosis on longevity, there has been a clear association between improvement in energy efficiency and therefore a reduction in food consumption. Also in a state of ketosis, it is easier to establish intermittent fasting. We already know that a caloric restriction extends life. We are beginning to see that intermittent fasting has a similar effect.

EPILEPSY

Ketogenic diets have long been used to mitigate neurological diseases such as epilepsy. In fact, it is considered one of the most effective interventions against this disease.

RISKS OF THE KETOGENIC DIET

The ketogenic diet does not have too many problems if it is done well.If you do not watch well to consume enough vegetables or other foods rich in micronutrients, a deficit of vitamins, minerals and fiber can be generated. This problem is easily avoidable if a varied diet is maintained and vegetable fat is obtained, such as avocado, nuts and leafy vegetable fiber.In this case, experts also recommend that vegetables always keep as much macro and micronutrients as possible. Therefore, depending on the vegetable or, eat it without cooking like arugula, or cook it at low temperature for hours.It is common to confuse low carbohydrate intake with high protein intake. Consuming too much protein activates the path of gluconeogenesis that transforms the amino acids of the protein into glucose and therefore we cannot get into ketosis.

The ketogenic diet is not advisable in people with liver or heart problems since in some cases it has led to the development of arrhythmias.

Diabetics also have to watch out for ketoacidosis, a state in which too low levels of insulin cause a buildup of ketone bodies that lower blood pH. This is quickly solved with good insulin control and is no problem for non-diabetic people.

The worst problem is the social pressure to eat carbohydrates. Surely many of those who already follow the Paleo diet will have experienced episodes of social rejection for not eating pasta. Imagine if we also restrict all carbohydrates!

METABOLIC FLEXIBILITY

I hope that with this book you have convinced yourself of the benefits of the ketogenic diet.This does not mean that now we all have to throw all the potatoes in the trash and only eat fat.One of the great evolutionary advantages that the human being has is its great adaptability and this includes our metabolism.Being metabolically flexible will give us the ability to adapt quickly to different situations, both consumption, and energy expenditure.Glucose is a good source of energy, which is why we like sweets and, in cases of anaerobic requirements, it is essential. Nor would it be good for excess ketosis to lose the ability to use it.Then you can alternate cycles of intake of different macronutrients.In the same way that our ancestors crowded with fruit during the summer to spend winters with canned and dried meat, we have to educate our body to be flexible to different diets.

PROPOSAL OF KETOGENIC DIET MENU

A ketogenic diet is strict on the subject of ingredients and consumption of macronutrients (carbohydrates, fats, and proteins) so it is always better for someone to guide you at the beginning until you have enough experience.

To maximize the benefit of the ketogenic diet we recommend:

- Drink lots of water or vegetable and bone broths.
- Do not increase protein intake (1.2-2 gr / kg body weight).
- Do not forget to train on an empty stomach, here you can see the benefits of training on an empty stomach.
- Make maximum 3 meals / day. Even if you can, reduce to 2.
- When the session is a HIIT, give it your all. We need the adrenaline to go up and your body to decide to mobilize the last savings (those under the mattress). Even if you like coffee you can have one to give that last push. You can add coconut oil to coffee (you will be fasting but you will eat the world).
- Rest and give yourself time to recover between sessions. If not, cortisol can play tricks on us.

07

KETOGENIC DIET AND HEALTH BENEFITS

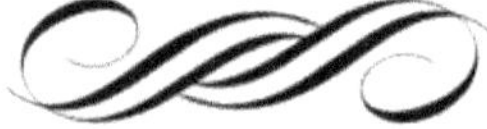

Promotes weight loss: This type of diet is designed to achieve a process called ketosis, that is, for the body itself to produce small molecules known as ketones, which are responsible for burning fat when eaten Very few carbohydrates and only moderate amounts of protein

2. Reduces acne: eating a diet rich in carbohydrates can alter intestinal bacteria and cause fluctuations in blood sugar, which also affects dermatologically. Therefore, by reducing your intake, you can reduce acne symptoms.

3. Improves cardiovascular health: Good cholesterol levels increase significantly, while bad cholesterol tends to decrease when this type of diet is followed.

4. It enhances the functioning of the brain: some studies show that this plan offers neuroprotective benefits so that it

can help prevent Parkinson's disease, Alzheimer's, or even sleep disorders.

5. Energizes the organism: it is believed that the combination of harrow, protein, and carbohydrates alters the way in which the body uses energy, enhancing and accelerating its ketosis process.

Optimize The Ketogenic Diet Through Your Digestive Health

Ketogenic diets are making a lot of noise, your friends have tried them, health coaches recommend them.

But what is it exactly? The ketogenic diet is one where you eat mostly fats, a little protein, and very few carbohydrates. There are several ways to do it but in general, in percentages, it would be like this: 75% fat, 20% protein, and 5% carbohydrates. Basically what happens is that the body goes into ketosis and uses fats as energy.

Why do people speak wonders of this type of diet? Many people have helped them lose weight, they feel much more energetic than before, they improve their mental health, among other benefits.But little is heard of how you can optimize your benefits. If you already decided, this article explains how to make your change to the ketogenic diet even more effective and that your efforts and determination are worthwhile.

One of the bases is to have a digestive system that is working at 100%. This is extremely important because if your digestive system is altered or if your intestinal flora is in imbalance, it will be much harder for your body to obtain adequate and sufficient nutrients. That your intestinal flora is in balance is a way to achieve it. The bacteria that form the intestinal flora are very important for digestion. helping to absorb fats properly, in addition to that they can also help the production of specific digestive enzymes for the digestion of fats.On the other hand, eating fewer carbohydrates can be very healthy, but the disadvantage is that it can be more difficult to obtain prebiotic fiber. So we recommend taking probiotics that contain prebiotics.Now, if your goal is to lose weight through a ketogenic diet, it will be very important to take probiotics since multiple studies show that an unbalanced intestinal flora can affect your basal metabolic rate (how many calories you burn when you are inactive), which would contribute to weight gain.Optimizing your ketogenic diet by taking probiotics + prebiotics will lead you to reach your goals in a faster and healthier way.

The Ketogenic Diet And Alcohol

The Ketogenic Diet in some of its stages allows you to drink a glass of dry wine, or a few milliliters of Whiskey or Champagne. But this is just a drink and has a determined level of diet. Considering also that there are people to whom drinking can cause liver damage, especially when they do it in excess.

The key to all this is represented by the moderation that a person should have when consuming alcohol. For example, in another diet such as the Mediterranean, it is allowed to accompany the food with a glass of red wine, without any problem.

Many doctors have considered that a glass of wine a day, plus a low carb diet, can help prevent heart disease and make people have a happier life. But in other diets, this consumption of alcohol delays weight loss, so it should not be a behavior to follow if you want to obtain the expected results with the diet.

A small amount of alcohol can be taken during the Ketogenic Diet, as long as the beverage consumed is low in carbohydrates. However, it is recommended that if it is observed that weight loss stops, or the person's metabolism is being affected, alcohol consumption should be stopped or it will be negative for their health.

Many people who have begun to diet, have discovered that she has helped them reduce not only the desire to consume sugar, but also have stopped consuming alcohol at the same time. This is due to the fact that their need or impulse has diminished since with the diet their sugar fluctuations have leveled off.

Cyclic Ketogenic Diet

To address this point of the Ketogenic Diet, we will consider some important aspects, such as the fact that people by decreasing their carbohydrate intake, increase the energy expenditure of their body. So now you burn more calories represented in fat, accumulated in your body.

Obesity is an evil that affects a large number of people and especially in regions where it is customary to make fast meals on the street, because their pace of work does not allow them to do it in their homes, especially at lunchtime, which at dinner time, they do it with copious dishes, to replenish everything they missed eating during the day.And this leads them to suffer from overweight problems since dinner is mainly a meal that should be quite light, because it is close to bedtime, and your body will not have time to burn the calories that are being provided.Cyclic ketosis is one of the diets considered throughout the world, because they are effective, but should not be followed for too long, only what is necessary to recover the desired flexibility and burn fat, lowering as a consequence of weight.

It is very similar to that made with intermittent fasting that we have seen in the 50-day diet, performed with cycles of five and two days. For this diet, the person for a few days is maintained with a low carbohydrate intake, which will then be changed to a cycle where many carbohydrates will be eaten. Seen from the numerical point this would be like this: low cycle with about 50 grams of carbohydrates a day; High cycle you can consume up to 600 grams of carbohydrates.

This is a diet that has been recommended for people who practice bodybuilding and many athletes who need to build their muscle mass. Therefore, with the cyclic diet, muscle glycogen is reduced, when there is a carbohydrate load. With this, athletes face their workouts properly.This is done in a way that before replenishing energy, it is trained to end all glycogen reserves, then it goes back to a reserve phase, where fat is reduced, and fed with protein and carbonhydrates. So people enjoy each cycle because in the part where they are allowed to eat carbohydrates, eat the foods they like, which are not going to accumulate as fats because they are using them during their workouts to replenish glycogen. Considering glycogen, the substance that is abundantly present both in our liver, as in all the muscles of the body and that is transformed into glucose (sugar) when the body needs it.

VEGETARIAN KETOGENIC DIET

This diet is so versatile that even in the case of vegetarian people they have solutions and plans to offer; For this, it has a diet that is based on fat intake as well as proteins but having as its source its plant origin.Vegetarian people already consume foods that are a source of vegetable fats, the only thing that should be done is to incorporate them in greater quantity into a Vegetarian Ketogenic Diet, although they are allowed to consume eggs and dairy products. Here are the foods allowed on this diet.

Allowed fats

The sources of fats used in the diet for vegetarians are egg yolks, cheeses, cream, nuts, avocado, coconut, olives, seeds such as sesame, chia or squash.In addition to that, they can season their meals with a wide variety of oils such as olive, coconut, palm, cod liver or sesame.

Allowed proteins

People who follow this diet can consume a series of proteins that are allowed such as egg whites, plain yogurt, cheeses that are white, dried fruits either consumed in whole grain form or by using their flours, in the preparation of creams.All products such as soybeans and their drifts are allowed with grains known as legumes, with foods such as peas, chickpeas, lentils, and beans.You can consume foods such as mushrooms, and vegetables such as spinach or broccoli, quinoa, both chia or pumpkin seeds, and some meat substitute used by vegetarians and called Tempeh, soy, Quorn, seitan, etc.The diet also allows the consumption of algae called spirulina, which is considered as an important source of both protein, vitamins and minerals, is not only food but also considered a dietary and nutritional supplement.

Vitamin supplements

People who make the Vegetarian Ketogenic Diet can consume both eggs and dairy products, as they need nutrients to maintain a good state of health since they are people who do not consume any type of meat.But when with the elements incorporated this vitamin contribution is not enough, it is necessary that vitamins and minerals be consumed independently, as they are necessary to keep your body functioning, thus avoiding the presence of diseases.It is important that vitamins such as B12, D, calcium and iron supplements be taken, which is usually obtained by eating meat, which vegetarian people do not realize, but can be consumed by dietary supplements that contain them.

Tips

Vegetarian people who want to start the Ketogenic diet are offered a series of suggestions, which are also very useful for many other people who can decide and follow these types of diets, these are the following:

- If you need to sweeten your drinks and food, you can do it with some kind of sweetener, not with sugar.
- To make meals more pleasant, the use of aromatic species is allowed.
- Vitamin supplements such as B12 and calcium should be available.
- For cases where carbohydrates are allowed they should not contain any type of starch.
- Not all fruits are allowed, in the case of the Vegetarian Ketogenic Diet the strawberry, raspberry, blackberries and strawberries are allowed.
- As for drinks, soft drinks without calories are allowed, as is tea or coffee, but they should always be taken without sugar.

The Ketogenic Diet as well as many other types of regimens that people usually follow, in order to lose weight, or perhaps only to cleanse toxins from their body and improve the way they feel. A series of risks may be associated, so before starting a dietary change it is necessary to consult with your doctor.

This type of diet is carried out in accordance with the weather, diets with respect to the allowed meals and avoiding those that are prohibited; It does not usually present any problem in general for people.

However, it can create some deficits of vitamins, minerals or fibers, since foods that are rich in these types of micronutrients are not present in their diet. For this, it is advised that the diet be carried out in a varied way with all the recommended food alternatives.

It is also necessary to consume fats of plant origin, such as avocado, drink coconut water, eat nuts and incorporate the fibers contained in leafy vegetables. In addition, high protein consumption should be avoided.Logically this is a type of diet that can be risky for people suffering from certain diseases, especially heart disease, hypertension, epilepsy, diabetes, and many others. Especially because they are people who are under medication programs, and whose physical condition is not normal.However, the final risk would be, the social problem, to call it in some way, because the people who are performing the Ketogenic Diet, when having a social gathering, where a series of dishes to taste are presented, should avoid consuming likewise, what is not allowed, however, can degenerate into social rejection.

Opinions about the Ketogenic Diet

Most experts in the field believe that with this type of Ketogenic Diet, the body becomes accustomed to all kinds of food, which will make it harder for it to gain weight again, especially in an exaggerated way.

It has established food plans that can be followed by people according to each of their particular needs, for example, if you only need to lose a few kilos of weight, the person can quietly just follow the plan for 10 days and with It will make you satisfied with your achievements.

But if on the contrary you have an overweight condition, before which you need a longer diet, you can choose to continue with that of 30 or 50 days, depending on your needs, all in its benefits and especially because of the fact that After having about 25 days with the diet, you can start an alternative diet and rest plan.

This final program of the Ketogenic Diet aims at the fact that the human body adapts to work properly and provide your body with energy, not only provided by carbohydrates, but also through the generation of ketosis, where He has learned to burn fat as a source of energy for his body.

Many people in the media give their opinions because they have already made these types of diets. Other opinions focus on nutritionists who have seen the progress made by their patients undergoing this type of diet.

All of them manifest and agree on the fact that if a person decides to go on a diet they should concentrate on it and do it well. For this, there are many menu options as well as many modalities of this diet, which allow you to choose the one that best suits your personal condition.

You can lose weight with it, without starving, at least it is what most people say; which consider that the worst stage is the initial stage, but once the body gets used, like people mentally everything goes easier.

Food Education Risk On Ketogenic Diet

The ketogenic diet is a diet based on the reduction of carbohydrates with almost exclusive use of lipids and proteins. The importance of this diet, from the clinical point of view, can be traced back to the early 1920s when it began to be used in the treatment of drug-resistant epilepsy in children. The use, instead, in the treatment of obesity is had beginning from the seventies. This diet induces the body to produce ketone bodies (acetone, acetoacetate, and 3-hydroxybutyrate), the production of which occurs when a very low or zero amount of sugar is taken.

Our body enters a physiological state called ketosis, in which it begins to burn fat and to use ketone bodies for energy purposes. In addition, minimum levels of sugar control the concentration of insulin, preventing the accumulation of fat. It is generally expected to combine with supplements such as omega 3, whey protein, spirulina, and essential amino acids, to maintain a proper balance of macro and micronutrients.

The diet includes two phases: In the first phase, we will have the elimination of carbohydrates, in the second phase their reintegration, with a maximum duration of 12 weeks. It is highly contraindicated for pregnant and lactating women, those suffering from hepatic, cardiac, renal insufficiency, type 1 diabetes patients and people with mental disorders.

Generally the results are rapid but a diet of this kind involves great stress and side effects for the body; among the short-term, transient and easily manageable ones we find: increased risk of uremia due to overloading of the kidneys, loss of appetite, transient lethargy, acidosis, gastro-oesophageal reflux disease, nausea, and vomiting.

On the contrary, in the long-term effects, there are hair loss, xerostomia, constipation from the absence of fibrous foods, nephrolithiasis, hyperlipidemia, hypoglycemia with possible nervous system problems, biliary calculus with consequent surgical treatment through cholecystectomy.

This type of diet in some contexts can be particularly harmful, it should not be understood as a definitive diet because it is strongly unbalanced, if excessively restrictive it must be abandoned and replaced with other food plans. It is a method where the "do it yourself" is absolutely banned, where an accurate medical check is required in order to assess the balance between risks and benefits on the organism.

Food Happiness Passes Through Conscious Choices

The health and energy of our body depend above all on the quality of the foods we ingest. In spite of this, of all the substances that we take daily, most of them do not nourish the body but damage it.

Saturated fats, junk food, spirits, sugars, and refined flours act negatively on our body weakening it and exposing it to the risk of more or less worrying pathologies. Good prevention aims to keep our body healthy, thanks to daily choices that must not be rigid and inflexible and a series of attentions that we voluntarily decide to implement in our lives, choosing a balanced, varied and harmonious diet.

In 2003, the Ministry of Agricultural and Forestry Policies published the new "Guidelines for a healthy diet". These lines are a useful tool, since, with scientific clarity and depth, they provide us with practical tips to be adopted in everyday life to maintain and promote our state of health. The practical tips that we find in these guidelines are to increase the consumption of fruits, vegetables, legumes and cereals such as, bread, pasta, rice. This will allow our body to receive daily vitamins, mineral salts, fibers and proteins of vegetable origin. Fibers are important for good bowel function. We must try to keep body weight constant through a physical exercise that must be constant and moderate.

It is advisable to limit the use and quantity of saturated fats, which are divided into saturated fats of animal origin, such as butter and lard and fats of vegetable origin such as olive oil or oil derived from other seeds, and they are defined as unsaturated fats, which in turn differ in mono and polyunsaturated, in this case it is advisable to consume polyunsaturated fats and limit the use of monounsaturated fats. It is necessary to moderate the use of sweets and more generally of sugary drinks.

Excessive intake of these foods can favor the onset of problems related to an increase in weight and related diseases, such as obesity. Attention should be paid to the fact that cane sugar has the same energetic value as refined sugar and that "light" products still provide calories.

Among the recommendations, the issue of water consumption is also mentioned as our body is composed of approximately 75% of it, which is therefore fundamental and vital for maintaining our health. For an adult man, the requirement is about 1 ml of water for every kilocalorie coming from the foods of our diet.

It is also necessary to regularize the use of salt, which should be consumed in moderation. The main sources of sodium are table salt, sausages, cheeses, olives, peanuts. It is good to reduce their consumption because it is already naturally contained in many foods. At the table, the salt could be replaced by learning to cook and flavoring foods with aromatic herbs such as rosemary, thyme, marjoram, and sage.

The consumption of alcohol should also be reduced, bearing in mind that during the meal it is advisable not to exceed the consumption of wine, which should be around the glass and a half. Everything is connected to the fact that since we are children we are used to loading the foods we eat with emotional values, such as a nice piece of chocolate makes a difficult situation to deal with less "bitter", and an abundant portion of cake the cream helps us to soothe our sorrows.

Today there is an increasing tendency to indicate diets of all types: from sports diets to those for housewives, to the east or the zodiac sign. The pleasure of eating and the resulting well-being are for our organism the result of more elements and values such as biological and cultural. Ultimately, given the various and complex behavioral consequences associated with food, it becomes increasingly important to pay due attention to communicating the knowledge of right eating habits.

MISTAKES OF THE KETO DIET

1: THE DIY

The ketogenic diet should never be done on its own. It is a low-calorie regime in which calories, carbohydrates, fats, and proteins are calculated precisely so it is absolutely necessary to consult a professional who is able to adapt macronutrients to the various phases of the diet.

2: DO NOT DRINK OFF

When following a ketogenic diet it is necessary to drink more water than usual, at least 2 liters a day, to maintain adequate hydration. The reduction of carbohydrates, in fact, causes a reduction in body water, since glycogen binds to itself a considerable amount of water.

3: DO NOT TAKE MINERAL SALTS

The ketogenic diet reduces a series of foods with consequent mineral deficiency, so it is advisable to take supplements such as potassium, magnesium, and sodium.

4: ABANDON THE DIET

When the body starts to burn fat instead of sugar it goes into a state of ketosis. To make the body, and especially the central nervous system, keto-adapted, it is necessary that the concentration of ketone bodies is high and in general higher than 2/3 mmol / L in order to compete with glucose for entry into the brain. At this point, there is generally a feeling of energy both mental and physical. Before this metabolic passage, we must not be discouraged if we feel a normal state of exhaustion.

5: TAKE DRUGS CONTAINING SUGAR

Pay attention to the drugs used during a ketogenic diet because they could contain quantities of sugar that are going to negatively affect the diet. Pay attention therefore to ingredients such as fructose, sucrose, glucose, dextrose, maltodextrin, etc.

6: DO NOT VISIT US

The ketogenic diet must be started and pursued under medical supervision because it is absolutely necessary to take the right amount of nutrients. As far as proteins are concerned, for example, if less than the necessary ones are taken, there is a risk of muscle catabolism; if they are taken in greater quantities, they risk exiting from ketosis due to gluconeogenesis.

7: DO NOT PLAN MEALS

In the ketogenic diet, following a food plan is very important. Not planning meals leads to easy errors in the intake of macronutrients and therefore to an exit from ketosis.

Planning saves frustration and malaise and makes it possible to identify exactly the phases in which the diet passes.

8: MAKE COMPARISONS WITH OTHERS

There are so many factors that come into play and influence the results when one undertakes a diet for which it is not possible to make comparisons with other people. Not everyone gets the same results, or there may be similar but achieved results at different times.

9: TOUGH TOO MANY PROTEINS

During a ketogenic diet, the body uses fats as a fuel source and needs proteins to protect the lean mass. However, it is necessary to introduce the right dose of protein and it is therefore very important to have a tailor-made food plan. When you consume more protein than you need, you end up converting those proteins into glucose, which in turn can increase blood sugar levels and get you out of ketosis.

10: DON'T SLEEP ENOUGH

It is very important to allow the body to sleep and rest sufficiently in order to face another day full of energy. Lack of sleep can contribute to fatigue and therefore to finding unsuitable foods that supply energy quickly.

08

STRETCHES OF THE KETOGENIC DIET

When we talk about stretches of the Ketogenic Diet, we refer precisely to the stages that are followed during the realization of this type of diet during the thirty-day period, which we will expand later.

The diet is designed in the form of stretches represented by periods of 10 days each, were allowed and prohibited foods are indicated, in order for people to organize their menu, based on them, thus carrying out the entire diet, thereby They can lose weight quickly.

Which is estimated may be over 12 kilos, after the three sections established for it has been completed, and are the ones we will mention below:

Section 1

It is the hardest section to be the initial and most restrictive, where the person will take note of their weight, to establish the differences obtained during these first 10 days, in which the foods allowed to avoid boredom will be combined.

Section 2

When people reach this stretch, they begin to manifest weight loss, consumed for another 10 days allowed foods, with others that are incorporated into the diet.

Section 3

It is the section formed by the last 10 days of the plan, offering the possibility that in addition to the allowed foods, whole-wheat pasta can be consumed; and with the difference that on the 25th the diet is broken and eaten at will. Then follow the diet until you complete your 30 days.When this section is completed, a modality is presented, which is to take a break, and then carry out an intermittency plan, where some days are dieted and others are not. Which we have explained in detail in the 30-day Diet.

Does it have a rebound effect?

Most diets usually have a rebound effect, since certain foods that used to be consumed daily are suppressed in order to make a new eating plan that allows fat burning, and most of the time; When you leave the diet you gain weight again, which is called the rebound effect.But this diet offers a plan that is adopted for the 30-day diet as well as the 50-day diet, where people alternate diet and other free days where they consume all the carbohydrates they want, and so their body gets used to make use of both fats and carbohydrates, to supply energy contributions.However, a good measure after the experience that people have acquired through their diet, is that they change their eating habits as much as possible, thus avoiding suffering this so-called rebound effect.

When the diet begins, the foods that are allowed in it are established, so that it is effective and that a state of ketosis can be reached, which is the one that will promote the burning of body fat, being essential to avoid most of the Carbohydrates, for this you must consume foods that favor fat production.

Being the foods that provide these fats, butter, coconut oil, avocado, olive oil, nuts such as almonds, nuts, hazelnuts and many others that contain fat, but are considered soluble.In the diet, you can consume foods that are low in carbohydrates, at least, less than 5%, such as meat, eggs, fish, and vegetables, and you can also consume some protein, but very little.The liquids that must be consumed first is water, then coffee or tea, but without sugar; and lastly, red wine, because it has carbohydrate contributions. Sometimes you can consume milk moderately or cream.

On the otherhand,Foods that contain a lot of sugar or starch are prohibited in the Ketogenic diet. Considered of this type are foods represented by potatoes, rice, pasta, and bread. All this because very high in carbohydrates.

Other foods that present this condition are soft drinks and juices, chocolates, sweets, beer, candies, and most fruits, at least sugary ones. As it should be considered that carbohydrate contributions should not exceed 10%, for proteins a maximum of 25% is allowed and fats must provide 70% of their diet.

09

IS THE KETOGENIC DIET USEFUL FOR TREATING PAIN?

If we talk about the ketogenic diet, we could immediately think of the professional bodybuilder (or who thinks he is) who uses this dietary approach to lose weight, and then define himself, before the races or, simply, before doing the swimsuit test.

But the ketogenic diet was not actually born for this purpose. It was used in principle as a therapeutic approach for those children who suffered from epilepsy and, to date, is also used effectively to reduce migraine. But to date, studies on the ketogenic diet are expanding and attempts are being made to validate efficacy also in the management and treatment of chronic pain and fibromyalgia.

How was it guessed that the ketogenic diet reduced pain?

As mentioned, the first ketogenic diet protocol was used to treat children with severe episodes of epilepsy. It was noted that if these children were subjected to a forced fast, the convulsions decreased dramatically. Then one wondered how to insert a food program that could "mimic" the effects of fasting and thus be able to simulate the effect of real fasting and, consequently, reduce epileptic attacks. Therefore, although today it is used as a useful approach to weight loss, in reality, it was born as a medical treatment.

Today it is also used effectively for the treatment of metabolic syndromes, migraine, obesity, Parkinson's disease, dementia, Alzheimer's and pain.

Unfortunately, it should also be specified, as we have seen very well in the application of the ketogenic diet to chronic migraine, that the results in terms of efficacy are maximized during the period of caloric restriction, usually a month. Further studies are underway to try to formulate a dietary plan consistent with a long-term approach. Why specify application times? Because the ketogenic diet, if used for prolonged periods and without supervision, can be dangerous for the body.

How it works in general terms

The ketogenic diet, commonly known as Cheto or Keto (I think) is born as a diet rich in fats and low in carbohydrates although, in more recent times, it has been modified by further cutting the total calories by introducing a new approach used in the clinical setting: the very-low-calorie ketogenic diet. This calorie cut is based on the further reduction of calories introduced by fat. Since these are an important caloric source, it was decided to stabilize them on a dosage of about 10-20 g per day. Being low in fat and carbohydrates, it is self-evident that the greatest caloric intake comes from proteins.By minimizing the explanation of how the ketogenic diet works, we could say that our body needs energy, an energy that is produced through food intake to function. Normally, through our metabolism, we derive energy mainly from carbohydrates, while fats are normally "stored" as an energy reserve which, if in excess, allows us to entertain our partner with our "love handles" .

Seriously, if this caloric intake decreases drastically, as in fasting, our body goes in red code, in alarm. The ketogenic diet actually simulates an illusion of fasting and, therefore, sets in motion the same alarm mechanisms. This alarm is activated through two mechanisms: reduction of caloric intake and reduction of carbohydrates, which represent the main source of "immediate use" energy.

How it works in detail

The fat. Our flesh we hate so much is actually (small consolation) our biggest energy reserve. Carbohydrate stocks, our "ready to use" energy, is definitely very paltry instead. The sugar reserves, in fact, can guarantee energy only for very limited periods. Obviously, if present, the body prefers them, but when it is scarce our body can also use fatty acids as an energy source or it can even convert some amino acids into glucose through gluconeogenesis.

However, some structures, among which our nervous system, are not able to use fatty acids, ama are however able to use ketone bodies, substances derived from stocks of fat (lipids), whose concentration in normal conditions it's almost nothing.

In the case of fasting or a ketogenic diet, the ketone bodies dramatically increase in number, sending the body into a condition of ketosis, a natural process that allows us (it would be more appropriate to talk to the past in the West and say it allowed) to survive in the absence of food. But the same condition also occurs after important physical efforts or in the morning.

The reduction of carbohydrates, through indirect action on insulin and glucagon, promotes lipid mobilization from our reserves in order to use them for energy purposes, through the production of ketone bodies. These are the perfect fuel to also nourish the functions of the central nervous system.This metabolic state is called ketosis and, as long as it remains within certain limits, it is physiological. Physiological ketosis does not contribute to changing the pH which, although it decreases slightly during the first days of the diet, returns to normal limits to stabilize. This until the concentration of ketone bodies remains at the standard levels that settle below 10 mmol / l.

Ketosis, by modifying the concentrations of certain hormones and substances, including leptin, ghrelin and the ketone bodies themselves, also allows the reduction and, in some cases, the disappearance of the sensation of hunger associated with ketosis.

Ketosis is not ketoacidosis

Physiological ketosis should not be confused with ketoacidosis associated with diabetes. This is an extremely serious condition that can potentially lead to death. It develops in people with type 1 diabetes due to a prolonged lack of insulin intake. This condition produces an increase in ketone bodies above 25 mmol / l with a total inability to properly dispose of them. This phenomenon allows a reduction in pH that can fall below 7.3, which, of course, can lead to death.

Nutrition for the sportsman is essential, a factor that together with training and rest is able to influence in a decisive way quality and level of performance. Ketogenic diet and sports may seem a not too convincing combination, at least on paper, but a good number of recent studies show that this type of diet can have really interesting applications in the sports field.

The ketogenic diet is a diet characterized by very low carbohydrate intake, below 30 grams per day, with a normal protein intake and a marked increase in fat consumption. A diet of this type determines some important changes in the use of energy substrates: within a few days, the reduced availability of carbohydrates causes the body to exhaust its glycogen reserves and start using fatty acids and ketone bodies, the latter produced in the liver from fatty acids.

In an adapted subject, after two or three weeks of diet, the fatty acids become the preferred substrate at the level of the muscle while the ketone bodies are destined to satisfy the energy demands of the central nervous system, which cannot use the free fatty acids incapable of cross the blood-brain barrier, along with a modest amount of sugar produced in the liver from some amino acids, glycerol, and lactic acid.

A ketogenic diet determines a whole series of adaptations at the level of the various organs and tissues which, substantially, predispose the organism to the use of lipids as a preferential energy source. At the same time, if the protein intake is well-calibrated, there is no loss of muscle mass, unfortunately very frequent in other diet models.

During a ketogenic diet the body enters a physiological state of ketosis, with an increase in the blood concentration of ketone bodies - usually less than 0.1 mmol / L - up to 7-8 mmol / L, without significant alterations of parameters fundamentals such as blood glucose and blood pH. Ketosis can be considered an important adaptive mechanism to situations of reduced food availability, a mechanism that is even more important in humans, given the close dependence of central nervous system functions, which alone accounts for over 20% of energy expenditure daily, from the availability of a certain amount of glucose.

The ketogenic diet is widely used in the therapy of a whole series of pathologies, starting from childhood epilepsy, and is increasingly popular as a weight loss diet. It is a well-studied protocol, which presents interesting advantages and whose side effects are well known and avoidable, with the necessary precautions.

CONCLUSIONS

Once you know what ketosis is and how it acts on the body, it is easier to understand why the ketogenic diet helps you lose weight steadily and steadily. Although the ketogenic weight loss diet has its advantages and disadvantages, it is a plan that meets the expectations of those who wish to lose weight and do so effectively.

However, the recommendation is that to follow the ketogenic diet, medical control is necessary, as it is a nutritional plan restricted in vitamins, minerals and low presence of fibre.

For those who want results in a short time, the ketogenic diet to lose weight can meet your expectations, but if you are looking to change lifestyle and eating habits, the option that nutritionists recommend is a plan to achieve higher longevity. In the long run, it is best to have a well-balanced, personalized diet where nutrients are lacking.

www.ingramcontent.com/pod-product-compliance
Lightning Source LLC
Chambersburg PA
CBHW061355250726
48657CB00004B/1504